An Orientation to Hospitals and Community Agencies

Joellen W. Hawkins, R.N.C., Ph.D., F.A.A.N., a professor at Boston College, serves as coordinator for the MCH tract in the Graduate Program in Nursing. She obtained a master's degree in maternal child health nursing, and a Ph.D. from Boston College, and has extensive clinical experience in obstetrics/gynecology/women's health as well as serving on the faculties of Salve Regina College and the University of Connecticut. She has taught undergraduate students for their first experience in a hospital and in ambulatory settings as well. She has written or collaborated on more than a dozen books and more than two dozen articles, and has contributed chapters to three books. Her books include *Clinical Experiences in Collegiate Nursing Education, Nursing and the American Health Care Delivery System,* and *Postpartum Nursing Health Care of Women.*

Evelyn R. Hayes, R.N., Ph.D., is Chairperson, Department of Nursing Science, College of Nursing, University of Delaware. Her practice area is community health nursing. She obtained a master's degree in community health nursing at the University of North Carolina, School of Public Health, and a Ph.D. at Boston College, and has worked in community health and taught at the University of Connecticut School of Nursing. She has taught undergraduate students at all levels of the curriculum, including first experiences in community health agencies, as well as serving as coordinator and faculty member for a graduate program in community health nursing. She has written and collaborated on several articles, contributed chapters to several books, including *Curriculum Development From a Nursing Model,* and presented research and scholarly papers at local, regional, national, and international meetings.

Cynthia S. Aber, R.N., M.S., Ed.M., is an Instructor at Boston College School of Nursing. Her expertise in practice is in maternal child health. She earned a master's degree in maternal child health nursing and a master's in health education at Boston University, where she is presently a student in a doctoral program. She has extensive clinical experience as a staff nurse and head nurse and has taught on the faculties of Lasell Junior College and Simmons College. For a number of years, she has been teaching students beginning their clinical experiences in hospitals. She is widely known as a master teacher.

An Orientation to Hospitals and Community Agencies

Joellen W. Hawkins, R.N.C., Ph.D., F.A.A.N.
Evelyn R. Hayes, R.N., Ph.D.
Cynthia S. Aber, R.N., M.S., Ed.M.

SPRINGER PUBLISHING COMPANY
New York

Springer Publishing Company, Inc.
536 Broadway
New York, NY 10012

86 87 88 89 90 / 5 4 3 2 1

Library of Congress Cataloging-in-Publication Data

Hawkins, Joellen Watson.
   An orientation to the hospital and community agencies.
   Bibliography: p. 145
   Includes index.
   1. Nursing—Social aspects. 2. Hospitals—Sociological aspects.
3. Community health services—Sociological aspects. I. Hayes, Ev-
elyn R. II. Aber, Cynthia S. III. Title. [DNLM: 1. Community
Health Services—organization & administration—United States. 2.
Hospital Administration—United States. WX 150 H393o]
RA965.H38   1986   362.1′1′068   86-10040
ISBN 0-8261-5280-5 (soft)

Printed in the United States of America

Contents

Preface

This book is designed as an introduction to institutions in which you, as students in nursing and other health care professions, will learn the clinical practice skills and apply the theoretical knowledge of your professions in caring for patients. The hospital can be an anxiety-producing place for those about to begin their clinical experiences. The abbreviations and acronyms used to denote places and events within the hospital are more complicated and confusing than need be. Knowing what these mean can help clear up some of the mystery and assist you in becoming comfortable in a hospital setting.

Hospitals bombard your senses: paging systems; codes for fire safety; musak piped over the air; patient call buttons, patient emergency bathroom buttons; monitors; machines; the smells of food, medications, cleaning solutions; the laboratory; x-ray developing; the operating suite; and the sight of unfamiliar equipment, supplies, and furnishings; personnel and patients dressed in unusual clothing; and mysterious departments and services. Just as you will soon learn what the names and abbreviations mean within the hospital, so too you will learn the meaning of the sounds, sights, and smells that characterize a hospital.

Community health agencies and community-based health care services will present you with another whole set of clinical settings where nurses and other health care professionals work and where you, as students, will gain some of your clinical experiences. In the pages to follow, we will also explore and explain the names, abbreviations, and characteristics of these important health care settings.

We hope that reading this book will help make your clinical experiences more rewarding and less threatening, help you feel more confident and be more competent, and that you will have some understanding of how your profession fits into the hospital and community agencies and how these institutions fit into the larger health care delivery system.

Acknowledgments

To our students, without whom this book would never have been written; to our colleagues for their invaluable support and assistance; and to our families and friends who support us through project after project, what can we say but thank you.

To Dr. Springer for her ideas and for her faith in our ability, we are grateful, but more especially for her characteristics as a publisher with whom it is truly a joy to work. To Ruth Chasek, Nursing Editor at Springer, thank you for your confidence in us and your quiet support.

1

The Hospital

During your years as a student and as a member of a health care profession, you will spend at least some of your time in one or more hospitals. In this chapter, we will discuss the hospital from a variety of perspectives: administration, patient care services, and support services. Hospitals, just like other institutions in our society, vary in their organizational structure; their physical facilities; the services they offer to consumers; the individuals they employ; the manner in which they deliver services; their underlying philosophy and purpose; and their relationships with the community at large. Not everything you read in this chapter, therefore, will be applicable to every hospital; it is also possible that you will fulfill your entire career as a nurse without being aware of some of the hospital characteristics that we describe. We hope to provide you with enough data about variations of hospital characteristics and a sufficient number of examples so that you will know about these institutions before or during your first clinical experiences in them.

STRUCTURE AND ORGANIZATION

The organizational structure of a hospital reflects its sources of support; the community which sponsors it and whom it serves; its mission to the community; its fiscal structure (for-profit or nonprofit) and its sources of monetary support; the persons it employs; and the extent of its physical plant. In the discussion that follows, we will begin with the top of the organizational chart and work down, describing the structural and organizational characteristics that hospitals may have and the variations which exist among the thousands of institutions that call themselves hospitals in the U.S.A. (see appendices for examples of organizational charts).

Administration

Most hospitals are governed by a board of trustees. These trustees are either appointed and/or elected by the hospital corporation (or whatever corporate structure exists, be it nonprofit or for-profit) and serve for a specified number of years. The trustees represent the community at large and assist in the overall maintenance of and functioning of the hospital organization. Trustees are generally divided into committees set up to meet the needs of the individual institution, and individual trustees are chosen for the specific committees based on their backgrounds and expertise. For example, a trustee who is a bank officer would probably be a member of the finance committee, whereas the head of a construction company would be selected for the building committee.

Within the hospital structure, there is a much larger group, the members of the hospital corporation, who have a vested interest in the hospital in one way or another. These persons may include some physicians, nurses, members of the hospital auxiliary; citizens from the community at large; members of religious or ethnic organizations (especially if the hospital is run by a religious group, such as an order of nuns; a Protestant denomination; or an organization of members of a particular ethnic or cultural group); and local, state, or federal officials (if the hospital is supported by public money). In hospitals with a religious affiliation and/or ownership, there may be a slightly different structure with the religious order, the archdiocese, the denomination, or group as the governing body followed by a board of directors and a chief administrative officer. The composition of the corporation varies from institution to institution; what is important is that it does exist for virtually every hospital in this country as an important component of the administrative superstructure, responsible in a general way for the continued existence and operation of the hospital.

The chief executive officer (CEO in management language) of the hospital may be referred to as the administrator, the general director, or the president of the corporation. Under the hallmark of the administration are the various vice presidents, assistant administrators, department heads, or whatever corporate structure titling is in place. These administrators will vary in number and title, depending upon the size and complexity of the hospital, and are largely responsible for the day-to-day operations. To give an example, a large hospital could have the following: directors of development, fiscal services, personnel, planning and marketing, human resources, nursing services, patient services, pastoral services, infection control, social services, public affairs, community relations, finance, physical plant or facilities, and engineering. Or the hospital could have a simpler structure, with department heads in these areas: admitting, dietary, fiscal, housekeeping, maintenance, laboratory, ministry, pharmacy, medical records, public relations, nursing services, security, social services, purchasing, quality assurance, and telecommunications.

Another group within hospital organizations that might be characterized as administration are the chiefs of the various services. These might include: medicine, surgery, anesthesia, pathology, radiology, and any of the specialty areas of the particular institution, such as obstetrics and gynecology, neonatology, pediatrics, orthopedics, neurology, family medicine, and on and on.

The administrative area of particular interest to nurses is the organizational structure and hierarchy for nursing services. Here again, there can be variation among hospitals, particularly if there is a school of nursing associated with the hospital. The chief administrative officer for nursing is called the director of nursing services, vice president for nursing or for nursing services, the assistant administrator for nursing or for patient care services, the chief of nursing, and variations on these titles, depending upon the particular hospital structure and administrative nomenclature. There are generally one or more associate or assistant directors of nursing or clinical directors, followed by clinical coordinators or supervisors for all areas in which nursing care is delivered and for all three shifts, accounting for 24 hours a day, 7 days a week. It is important to remember that nursing is a service provided in hospitals 24 hours a day and, as such, requires the appropriate administrative superstructure to oversee delivery of care around the clock. The next level of administrative structure in nursing may be designated as nurse leaders, head nurses, nurse coordinators, or patient care coordinators for particular specialty areas such as medical, surgical, obstetric and gynecological, pediatric, and so on, depending upon the specialty services offered. Those individuals providing the most direct patient care are registered nurses (who may possess a diploma, associate degree, baccalaureate, master's or doctoral degree in nursing, or one or more degrees in another field), licensed practical or vocational nurses, and nursing assistants (aides and orderlies).

Hospitals vary in their employment of nursing personnel from selection of only one group, such as nurses with a minimum of baccalaureate preparation in nursing, to a wide variety of preparation from education to professional, vocational, or technical, and on-the-job training (aides and orderlies or nursing assistants or technicians). Decisions about the level of preparation necessary to deliver nursing care are based on the philosophy and objectives of the nursing department; the types of patient care services offered; the types of patients cared for; and the practice of nursing in the hospital. In the next section, we will discuss the provision of services to patients and the delivery of nursing care in the hospital setting.

PATIENT CARE SERVICES

The hospital is the primary setting for the acute care of patients in the U.S.A. Each hospital has its own philosophy, a general statement of its intention to deliver care and what its primary goal is to be: service to the community; teaching of health care professionals such as physicians and nurses; profit making for the corporation or stockholders; service to a particular group of individuals, such as veterans of military services or the indigent; or a combination of these. For example, most if not all teaching hospitals have a dual commitment: service to the community and the preparation of qualified health care professionals. These so-called teaching hospitals also often deliver primary care to individuals in the surrounding geographic community, as well as serving as specialty referral centers for the seriously ill and those with complex illnesses from around the country and the world.

The primary objective of any hospital is to provide care for the sick. Another basic objective might be to provide a clinical setting for the education of those responsible for delivering that care, even if the hospital is not designated as a teaching hospital. Yet another objective might be research into diseases, in the endless quest for answers to the questions of cause and cure. These objectives are representative of many hospitals.

Hospitals affiliated with a medical school are often referred to as teaching hospitals. What this means to a patient is that, in addition to his/her personal physician responsible for care, there is also a house staff of medical students, interns, and residents providing care and coverage when the personal or "attending" physician is not in the hospital.

Part of the daily routine in hospitals is for the residents, interns, medical students, and/or attending physicians to go on "rounds" to examine patients and discuss their individual medical treatment plans. Nurses may be included in these "rounds" and/or may conduct their own reviews of patient care. In institutions without house staff, the attending physician may make rounds alone or with a nurse to discuss his/her patients and modify or validate the medical plan of care.

Nursing care is the responsibility of the nursing staff, and is under the direction of a registered nurse when other nursing personnel are present. There are several ways of delivering nursing care. Team nursing means that a group of nursing personnel acts as a team to provide care for a group of patients and may divide up that care by tasks to be accomplished; by the complexity of care required by patients; and/or by patient assignments to each member of the team. Several variations on this form of organization exist. There is generally a team leader and several team members and usually two or more teams for a given unit or floor of patients. The head nurse or designate assumes responsibility for the overall functioning of the unit during a particular "shift" (period of working time that may vary from 8 to 10 hours).

Primary nursing is a term used to describe a specific way of delivering care and is being adopted by many hospitals. Primary nursing means that one nurse is totally responsible for the assessment, planning, implementation, and evaluation of a patient's care for a 24-hour period. The primary nurse oversees the nursing care whether she/he is actually the care provider or the care is given by an associate nurse when the primary nurse is not at work. This personalized way of delivering care gives patients access to one nurse and increases the nurse's accountability for the delivery of care to patients. Primary nurses are often actively involved in all care decisions, including the decision to discharge the patient and the planning that must be done before the patient goes home.

In addition to acute care inpatient services, a hospital might also have outpatient or ambulatory services. These may include a 24-hour a day emergency unit standing vigilant to serve any and all emergencies that occur, varying from a minor injury to a heart attack, rape or child abuse, substance overdose, or attempted suicide. The large number of patients seen in emergency rooms or departments is startling: some hospitals treat more than 50,000 patients a year.

Because individuals without a personal physician sometimes use emergency departments as their primary care providers, some hospitals have established separate walk-in services available up to 24 hours a day, 7 days a week to care for persons with upper respiratory infections, gastrointestinal upsets, ear infections, and other acute non-life-threatening illnesses or occurrences that are not really emergencies but do require somewhat immediate care to relieve the person's discomfort. Sometimes these units operate with limited hours, such as 8 a.m. to 6 p.m., and then the emergency department takes over. Some hospitals have primary care centers in addition to walk-in services. These function as primary care providers, and one can make an appointment just as one might with a private physician, nurse practitioner, or clinic. This service is especially treasured by newcomers to the community.

Hospitals often provide a variety of other ambulatory services, but these will be discussed in later chapters. By and large, hospitals exist first of all to provide acute care inpatient services and sometimes outpatient ambulatory services to those for whom care in other settings such as private physicians' offices, Health Maintenance Organizations (HMOs), freestanding clinics, community agencies, and the home is either inappropriate, inaccessible, or unavailable. In the next section of this chapter, we will discuss support services that are necessary to, but not directly involved with, the provision of care.

Support Services

In addition to the services that have already been discussed and those that will be discussed in detail in later chapters, there are many support services that are necessary to the smooth functioning of a hospital. These support services often go unnoticed, but it is because of their existence that hospitals can deliver to the consumer all we have come to expect. The support services include everything from the maintenance of the physical plant to the availability of oxygen when it is needed. Who is responsible for seeing that the oxygen supply is adequate, whether it is piped through the walls or delivered in tanks? The often unsung heroes and heroines of the hospital are those persons who provide support services such as the supply of oxygen so that we nurses can do our job of providing hands-on care to patients.

The *maintenance department* is an example whose services are quite broad and diverse, and yet essential to the smooth operation of the hospital. Many of us take for granted the impeccably clean floor; mattress replacement; maintenance of fire equipment; upgrading and repair of portable and fixed equipment; replacement of light bulbs; and the care of the thousands of mechanical items within the hospital, including the heating system and climate control. Where would any of us be without this support service to help in running a patient care facility?

The *dietary department* is another vital support service. At no other time than during illness does the body have such a need for healing nutrients. Insuring that the nutritional needs of an individual are being met, while also recognizing individual tastes, and restrictions, and attempting to serve attractive, palatable trays of food for large numbers of people is an awesome task for any dietary service. The diversity of tastes and the broad range of therapeutic diets needed daily is a challenge. Even restaurants are not faced with such demands. In a restaurant, the chef can employ techniques that will tempt the palate such as the use of cream, salt, spices, deep fat frying, and so on that are not always considered healthy practices. The hospital dietary department must make food appeal to patients while staying within the limitations of therapeutic diets. All meals must be calibrated to include the essential nutrients to promote healing and wellness, yet must be tasty and appealing to the eye or they will be returned untouched. Professional dieticians work in this department. These persons are involved in direct care of patients when planning diets and teaching about special dietary needs. They may be included in patient care conferences when the wellbeing of the patients is related to special dietary needs or modifications.

Central supply is an area that most consumers are unaware of. It is in this department where all sterilizing or autoclaving of materials or reusable supplies and materials is done. It is the responsibility of the personnel in central supply to provide all the equipment that the patient care units require, ranging from bedpans and bath basins to syringes and needles. So much of the equipment that hospitals use today is disposable that one can easily forget that an adequate supply of these items must be maintained. Central supply also stocks or can obtain special items needed for patient care that are not supplied on the nursing units or wards, such as small caliber urinary catheters and suture removal sets. Some hospitals have all supplies, disposable or reusable, processed by central supply and designate responsibility for all supplies used on nursing units to this department. In other institutions, central supply may perform some of the functions of providing supplies and others may be delegated to housekeeping, purchasing, and so on. Since patients are charged for many of the items used in their care, nurses may have to fill out charge cards and maintain records for supplies used. Delivery of items to nursing units occurs in a variety of ways. Sometimes a member of the central supply staff will visit the nursing units with a cart or basket to check and replenish supplies. In other institutions, a conveyor belt or dumbwaiter is used. Nurses need to know what equipment and services central supply provides, how to obtain items, and how to do the paperwork necessary for transactions.

The *purchasing department* has the responsibility for buying the supplies and equipment that the hospital requires, ranging from paper goods to machines. Sometimes this responsibility is shared with other departments, such as central supply, dietary, laundry, and maintenance. With all the new products being developed for hospitals, this department has the responsibility to choose the kind of equipment and the supplies that will be purchased that will keep costs down and at the same time replace outdated items.

The provision of all the linens required in a hospital is the responsibility of the *laundry or the linen room*. This department resembles a large linen closet with all the linens the hospital uses sorted in it. This linen usually includes sheets and pillowcases, blankets and spreads, draw sheets, hospital gowns for patients called "johnnys," flannel bath blankets, robes, towels, face cloths, and baby shirts and blankets. There are also isolation gowns and face masks, all the linens needed in the surgical suites and the delivery rooms, and the special attire worn by personnel in certain areas, such as scrub suits and dresses and surgical cover gowns. Disposable items have replaced some of these in some hospitals.

In recent years, while some hospitals have retained their own laundries, many have abandoned them in favor of getting linen supplied by a central agency that delivers to several hospitals. Some hospitals have joined together to support a central hospital laundry which then supplies all the member institutions. These practices have become more common than retaining the individual laundry and have been found to be cost-effective. Patients and staff members are usually unaware of whether the linen is being laundered and supplied within the hospital or from an outside agency. In the past, hospital laundries repaired the linens, cared for the uniforms of student nurses from the hospital school of nursing, and even made some items!

The *blood bank* is a department that is sometimes a part of the laboratory services. It is here that all the blood needs for the hospital are met. This department is responsible for typing and cross-matching of blood and the filling of the need for whole blood, plasma, platelets, packed cells, and any other blood products or components. Major surgery would not be possible if there were not an adequate supply of blood products available within the hospital. The blood bank also has to procure blood either through donors in the hospital or community or in cooperation with the Red Cross and other blood banks. This is one department that most consumers are aware of, as they often serve as donors.

The *pharmacy* is a department much like any community drugstore, but with a more serious mission and a less sundry orientation. The pharmacist is responsible for supplying all patients with all the medications they require during the hospital stay, as well as those they will take with them when discharged. Some hospital pharmacies also fill prescriptions for employees and for ambulatory and emergency room patients. This department may supply patient care units with syringes, needles, alcohol wipes, and any other items related to the administration of medications. It is also the responsibility of pharmacy personnel to replenish stock supplies of medications such as aspirin and laxatives on units, in medicine closets, rooms, or carts, and to supply solutions used to give care and clean patient areas, such as antiseptics and special hand soaps. Intravenous medications and solutions and the tubing also may come from the pharmacy. The pharmacist may mix medications for intravenous administration and also certain special medications, such as chemotherapeutics used to treat cancer. In some hospitals, a pharmacist visits each unit daily to check on the supply of medications for each patient. Many questions related to the administration or effects of drugs can be answered by the pharmacist. This department can be a much needed resource, given the constant flow of new medications on the market.

Personnel departments may be responsible for the recruitment, interviewing, hiring, retention, and firing of all personnel employed by the hospital, or this function may be decentralized so that nurses are hired by the department of nursing and so on. In addition to making sure that the hospital has all the persons necessary to carry on its work, the personnel department maintains records of all employees, does the paperwork required by the various benefits employees receive, and evaluates employee performance.

Public relations departments have played an increasingly important role for hospitals in recent years. Not only is the hospital part of the community, but it needs to inform the community about the diverse roles it plays. Publicity may be a responsibility of this department or a separate department may exist. In this age of technology, the public is interested in innovations in health care. Interacting with the media is an important support service that can enhance the hospital's status in the community, protect the privacy of patients, their families, and hospital personnel, and preserve or destroy the hospital's image.

As hospitals have become big businesses with huge budgets, multiple and complex sources of funding, many employees, and diverse needs for goods and services, the fiscal or accounting departments have become very important to everyday operations. Computers assist those responsible for the fiscal management of hospitals to do their jobs. Some hospitals have their own computers and others buy time on computers through time-sharing arrangements. Due to the increasing use of computers in hospitals, some institutions now have separate data processing or telecommunications departments.

The *record room* is an area critical to the operation of a hospital. It is here that all patient records are stored, once the patient has been discharged from the hospital. Should the patient be readmitted, the record can be retrieved so that those providing care can refer to the notes from the previous admission. One or more professional record librarians will probably staff the record room, in addition to secretarial staff and other paraprofessionals. With the technology available now through computers and microfilm, records are often converted to these forms for storage after a period of several years.

A *medical and nursing library* is often part of a hospital. Here are kept the books and journals that will be helpful to professional staff members. This department is generally staffed with one or more professional librarians, in addition to secretaries and other paraprofessionals. Members of the professional staff can use the library for reference and for research.

The *social service department* exists to assist health care professionals and patients and their families to identify financial and other resources, as well as to make the transition from hospital to home or community-based intermediate care facility. This department may also offer one-to-one and group education or counseling sessions on topics ranging from choosing a nursing home to coping with adolescents.

Staff education is an important part of professional practice and responsibility in a hospital. In general, the differentiation between in-service education and continuing education is that the former focuses on knowledge and skills necessary to do one's job and the latter more broadly on professional development. Sessions vary from updating on procedures and equipment to topics more germane to career development, such as writing for publication. Institutions may offer only one kind of education or may choose to offer both. It is not uncommon for a hospital to have a staff education or in-service education department. Sometimes this department is also responsible for orientation of all new employees or of all professional employees.

Of course, in some hospitals there are support services that we have not discussed here, or the services are organized in a different way and given different names. For example, the maintenance department in some hospitals may be broken down into *engineering,* responsible for heat, light, electricity, and the functioning of large pieces of equipment; *housekeeping,* responsible for the cleanliness of the building; and *buildings and grounds,* responsible for the upkeep, but not cleanliness, of the hospital buildings and land. Linen supplies may be subsumed under *central supply.* The best rule of thumb is, when in doubt, ask. Study the organizational chart and see which services are provided by each department, and ask questions if there's something you don't understand.

In the next chapter, we will examine hospital structure from several other perspectives: *monetary support,* patient services and principal orientation. From simple beginnings, hospitals have now become complex fiscal corporate structures, relying for support on many sources. Whereas the acquisition of sufficient money to run a hospital is not ordinarily the responsibility of nursing, cost-consciousness is. Increasingly, we are being asked to demonstrate our worth and to be accountable for the services we provide. An understanding of how hospitals receive their monetary support is helpful, therefore, in planning ways to determine what nursing care is worth to patients and the revenue it generates for the hospital. Furthermore, services have expanded along with technology and the diversity of hospitals is reflected in part in their principal orientation as teaching, community service or commercial enterprises.

2
Types of Hospitals

There are several types of hospitals, depending upon the classification system one chooses to use. They may be categorized by form of monetary support (private nonprofit, for-profit, and local, state, or federal government); by the patient services they offer (general; specialty, such as pediatrics, psychiatry); and/or by the principal orientation, whether that be community service, teaching, or commercial enterprise. Of course, these categories are not mutually exclusive. A hospital could, for example, be a government-supported long-term institution whose principal aim is service to a select community. In this chapter, we will explore what is meant by the various classifications of hospitals and how they differ from one another (see Table 2.1).

MONETARY SUPPORT

Modern health care technology feeds on a vast array of sophisticated machinery and expert health care providers, both of which are found in hospitals. Hence, providers of health care as well as consumers are dependent upon these

TABLE 2.1 Categorization of Hospitals by Source of Financial Support[a]

Government	
Federal	Department of Defense Army, Navy, Air Force (77 in U.S.)[b] Veterans' Administration (172)[b] Department of Health and Human Services Indian Health Service, Public Health Service Hospitals, St. Elizabeth's, NIH Clinical Center, hospital for Hansen's disease, Louisiana Department of Justice Hospitals in federal prisons
State government	Long-term hospitals for psychiatric care, care of persons with physical and learning disabilities Short-term hospitals for psychiatric care, state university medical school hospitals, hospitals in state prisons
Local government	District, city, town, and county hospitals—long- and short-term care facilities hospitals for city prisons
Voluntary (nonprofit)	Religious groups Independent nonprofit corporations; often "community hospitals" Miscellaneous: private industries or corporations (such as a railroad, mining company, or a union); Shriners hospitals (fraternal organization; cooperatives
Proprietary (for-profit)	Individual ownership Partnership Privately held corporation Publicly traded corporation

[a] Adapted from Wilson, F.A. & D. Neuhauser (1982). *Health Services in the United States.* Cambridge, MA: Ballinger, p. 9.
[b] Number of hospitals.

institutions. Dating from the church and monastery related hostels and hospices of the Middle Ages, the modern hospital still purports to offer a refuge to the ill. Confronted with the vast edifices of steel and concrete that we have come to know as hospitals, it is sometimes difficult to differentiate these health *care* institutions from other large corporations, however. Technology, advances in medical science, and the evolution of nursing as an educated profession have contributed to the changing image of hospitals that we have experienced in the 20th century. Whatever the reasons, hospitals have emerged, rightly or wrongly, as major institutions in the complex health care system in this country. They hold a monopoly on technology, often serving as the sole provider of certain types of diagnostic and therapeutic services. At the same time, the U.S.A. is struggling to contain the cost of health care, beset by an escalation in spending out of proportion to inflation. By examining the ways in which hospitals receive their monetary support, we may better understand why health care costs so much.

There are three major types of hospitals when one considers sources of financial support: private, nonprofit; government; and proprietary or for-profit. Of course, none of these categories exists in isolation from the other two.

Nonprofit Hospitals

In 1981, slightly more than half the hospitals in the United States were private and nonprofit, and over 80% of community hospitals were nonprofit (Statistical Abstract, 1984). Private, nonprofit hospitals are generally governed by a nonprofit corporation with a board of trustees from the community served. Sources of revenue for these hospitals include payments made directly by patients for services received (known as fee-for-service), reimbursement by a third party (Blue Cross, private insurance companies, government money through programs such as Medicaid and Medicare), or through special funds for indigent patients with no other means to pay. Some community hospitals receive support to provide "free" services through donations, endowments, special gifts, and sometimes arrangements with the community in which the hospital is located (see appendix for comparisons of Blue Cross/Blue Shield and private insurance and Medicaid and Medicare).

The term nonprofit means just that. At the end of a fiscal year, the hospital must show that any income generated in excess of expenses has been turned over into improvements of the physical plant, or services offered, or in some way accounted for other than as profit to the corporation.

Nonprofit community hospitals were often built originally with money raised by the community or through the generosity of wealthy benefactors. Today, many of these institutions must rely on patient fees and third-party reimbursement for their survival. Some are fortunate enough to have endowments or continue to have philanthropic members of the community dedicated to helping these institutions survive. Additionally, some rely on fundraising for their ongoing expenses and/or special projects, such as new equipment or construction. In 1946, the original Hill–Burton legislation was passed, providing money for hospital construction. Many community hospitals have been able to update their facilities with federal money under this bill and its amendments.

Hospitals Supported by the Government

Government supported hospitals have a long history, beginning with the hospitals, such as they were, that were founded in the 17th century to serve soldiers and the public almshouses that had infirmaries. Today, about one-third of short-stay hospitals are supported by local, state, or federal governments and there is a declining number of long-term hospitals, also government supported, most of which are psychiatric facilities. There are several categories of publicly supported hospitals: general hospitals that serve a given community; specialty hospitals, also serving a defined target population; general and specialty hospitals for those meeting special criteria, such as military hospitals for those on active duty, retirees, and dependents; the hospitals that form the network of the Veterans Administration; the federal hospital for Hansen's disease (leprosy) in Louisiana; the federal psychiatric hospital, St. Elizabeth's, in the District of Columbia; the National Institutes of Health Clinical Center in Bethesda, Maryland; hospitals that are part of the Indian Health Service; and the network of public health hospitals, the latter of which are slated to be closed in the 1980s. Each of these will be discussed in turn.

Local communities may have hospitals supported through public money to serve the population of the legally defined community. These hospitals are declining in number in response to escalating costs and the need for support from fee-for-service and third-party, as opposed to general tax, revenues. In the Northeast, local public hospitals generally serve a town or city. In the Midwest, South, and West where the county structure in government is active, there may be a county hospital serving the communities within its borders. State hospitals are supported, as their name suggests, by revenues generated by the state government, but they have come to rely more heavily in recent years on money from the federal government in the form of Medicare and Medicaid reimbursement. State hospitals tend to be specialty institutions, notably psychiatric facilities. State institutions for tuberculosis are now a thing of the past, but once figured prominently in the budgets of state governments. As deinstitutionalization of mentally ill and learning disabled individuals has become an accepted alternative to long-term institutional care, state hospitals have declined in number and size.

At one time, the federal government supported a network of public health hospitals, originally designed to serve the needs of seamen and of individuals struck down with communicable diseases. Under reorganization of the Department of Health and Human Services, these hospitals are being closed. The federal government plays a significant role in the direct provision of care through the military hospital system. Health services for the military are administered under the Department of Defense. The Navy has 23 stateside hospitals and medical centers, as well as 19 in U.S. territories and overseas. The Army has 48 hospitals and medical centers. The Air Force has six medical centers in the U.S.A. Through these hospitals and clinics, the federal government provides health care for 1) all military personnel on active duty and their dependents and survivors and 2) retirees and their dependents and survivors.

The Veterans Administration, founded in 1930, serves veterans of all the military services. Its health services arm consists of 172 medical centers across the country providing both general and specialty care.

The National Institutes of Health, the research arm of the Department of Health and Human Services of the federal government, operates a 500-bed clinical center in Bethesda, Maryland. Patients are referred from all over the country who are suffering from diseases currently under investigation by one or more of the research institutes.

The Indian Health Service, a federally funded entity, provides care for almost half a million native Americans and Alaskan natives through 51 hospitals, as well as health centers and clinics. Most of the hospitals in the contiguous 48 states are located on federal reservations.

The federal government is also responsible for two other hospitals: St. Elizabeth's, the federal psychiatric facility in the District of Columbia, and the national hospital for Hansen's Disease, (leprosy) located in Carville, Louisiana.

Thus, the role of government in providing care through the maintenance of hospitals at the local, state, and federal levels is extensive. Over the centuries of government involvement in hospital care in this country, however, the role has changed from one of widespread service to the population at large to care for selected groups of individuals.

Proprietary Hospitals

There are, in the United States, more than 900 hospitals operated on a proprietary basis or for-profit (Statistical Abstract, 1984, p. 113). The number is growing, as evidenced by reports in the papers announcing the purchase of hospitals by large corporations. As health care evolves from a philanthropic to a business orientation, it is likely that more institutions will be taken over by big corporations. For-profit hospitals, like any other businesses, are operated, as the name suggests, in order to show a profit for investment at the end of the fiscal year. Unlike nonprofit institutions, the corporate board and chief executive officer are under no obligation to reinvest profits in the institution, but may disperse them at their discretion. If shares for the corporation are traded on the open market, then the board is responsible to its shareholders, but not in a business sense to the community at large. There are two sides to this for-profit coin, however. Running a hospital like a business may offer the advantage of closer attention to cost containment and making sure that income more than covers expenses. On the other hand, a hospital is in the business of helping human beings, not producing a product or service far removed from life and death issues. There are those who would argue that the drive to generate a profit may in fact overshadow concern for human life and well-being. Of course, there are no simple answers to these complex questions. As health care providers, we have the responsibility to understand the type of institution in which we are practicing and examine the accountability of that institution for the mission in which it purports to engage.

There are some similarities between hospitals and hotels. The names, incidentally, come from the same root. The charges of each are based upon daily occupancy and, therefore, empty beds mean loss of money. Perhaps hospital charges should be calculated differently. Rates might vary depending upon the amount of care the patient requires, the diet, and so on. Hotels are much less expensive than hospitals and might even be used in conjunction with hospitals to keep costs down. The Children's Inn in Boston is adjacent to the Children's Hospital Medical Center. The Inn is a hotel where children and their parents can stay as an alternative to hospitalization when intensive nursing care on a 24-hour-a-day basis is not necessary, but when periodic assessments and treatments are required. This model might be used more extensively as an alternative. Hospitals, whatever the sources of funding, are very expensive institutions in our society and we would do well to explore any feasible changes or alternatives to help to provide the best possible care to those who need it at the best price.

BY PATIENT SERVICES

The services that hospitals provide to their patients may be loosely categorized as general, specialty, and long-term. What this means is that hospitals are in the business of providing residential care for patients with general acute care conditions, for those with special needs such as children and pregnant women, and for those requiring longer term care, but distinguished from nursing home or rehabilitation care. The services that a particular hospital can offer depend upon that hospital's geographic location, the needs and composition of the population it will serve, the health care professionals available to care for patients, and its physical facilities. A hospital in a rural area may provide general, specialty, and long-term care within the scope of its capabilities and staff, make referrals to other hospitals for special cases, and receive patients back from referral centers. An urban hospital close to other hospitals may offer highly specialized services or serve only a select population. In this section, we will discuss patient services under these three general categories, recognizing that they are neither mutually exclusive nor unique to any hospital.

General Patient Services

When describing most of the hospitals in this country, it is safe to say that they provide for the medical and surgical care of patients. What is meant by *medical care?* In this context, it refers to any care that comes under the heading of internal medicine. Any diseases or conditions that require the services of an internist or family practice physician come under this category (see Chapter 4 for discussion of physician specialties). If a patient is admitted for uncontrolled hypertension (high blood pressure) or for management of diabetes, he/she would be treated in a medical unit.

Under the heading of *surgical care* come all those conditions requiring the services of a general surgeon, from appendectomies to the repair of hernias. Specialty surgery by individuals prepared as ophthalmologists, thoracic surgeons, vascular surgeons, and so on may be done in community or general hospitals, and the patients may be admitted to general surgical units. In large hospitals, where the number of patients admitted for specialty surgery is great, there may be whole units devoted to caring for these patients. Surgery that is highly specialized, such as transplant surgery or cardiac surgery, is not often performed in community or small to moderate size (up to 300 beds) hospitals, but rather in medical center hospitals that have specialized patient care units with the skilled staff to care for patients pre- and postoperatively.

An area common to most hospitals is the *surgical suite.* In this department lie the operating rooms, pre-anesthesia or preoperative rooms, surgical supply rooms, and the recovery rooms for postoperative care.

There are usually several operating rooms, and to some extent, the number will depend on the size of the hospital and the amount of surgery done daily. Most operating rooms are in almost constant use from very early in the morning to late in the afternoon. Cases are usually scheduled from 7:00 a.m. to about 4:00 p.m. Emergency surgery may interrupt the schedule, but for the most part, the day shift handles most of the cases with just enough time for cleanup in between. With everything in the operating room being either tiled or made of stainless steel, the cleaning process can be completed in very short order in the interim between one case and the next.

When a patient comes to the surgical floor, he/she goes immediately to a holding area or a preoperative room. Final preparations are made here, such as starting the intravenous solutions and administering certain kinds of anesthesia. Caudal, epidural, and spinal anesthesia can be started in the preoperative area. Not every institution has a preoperative area or uses it for every surgical case, but many hospitals do have one to facilitate the smooth functioning of the operating suite.

After surgery, the patient is usually wheeled to the recovery room to recover from anesthesia and be monitored closely by the skilled nursing staff. The recovery room is located near the operating rooms and, should an emergency such as excess bleeding arise, the patient can be wheeled back into the operating room in a matter of seconds for treatment.

It is in the *recovery room* that a patient awakens from and/or recovers from anesthesia. The time spent here varies from patient to patient, and to some extent can depend upon the nature of the surgery performed and the type of anesthesia administered. The patient is not discharged from the recovery room until the vital signs are stable (blood pressure, pulse, respirations, temperature, and so on) and he/she is alert enough to respond verbally, such as being able to state her/his name.

Patients who require further skilled and vigilant monitoring after surgery will be moved from the recovery room to the intensive care unit. Most patients, however, once recovered from anesthesia and once vital signs are stable, return to their rooms on the surgical floor, where they are cared for by the nursing staff. In hospitals where primary nursing is practiced, it is likely that the primary nurse will assume postoperative care for the patient upon return to the unit.

Specialty Services

In addition to the medical and surgical units in a hospital, there may also be specialty areas. Most hospitals have at least one specialty unit, unless they are devoted to one specialty only, such as a psychiatric hospital.

The intensive care unit is one example of a specialty service common to many hospitals. The *intensive care unit (ICU)* is a specialized area fully equipped with state-of-the-art monitoring capabilities and a highly trained and experienced staff. Not all patients in the intensive care unit are necessarily surgical patients. There can be patients with medical diagnoses requiring intensive care as well. Many patients who have suffered myocardial infarctions (heart attacks) require even more monitoring and intensive care than those who have undergone a surgical procedure. Some hospitals have a special *cardiac intensive care unit (CICU)* to care for these patients who may require telemetry or cardiac monitoring, but others have only one intensive care unit to provide these services. Some hospitals have a *medical intensive care unit (MICU),* a *surgical intensive care unit (SICU),* and a cardiac

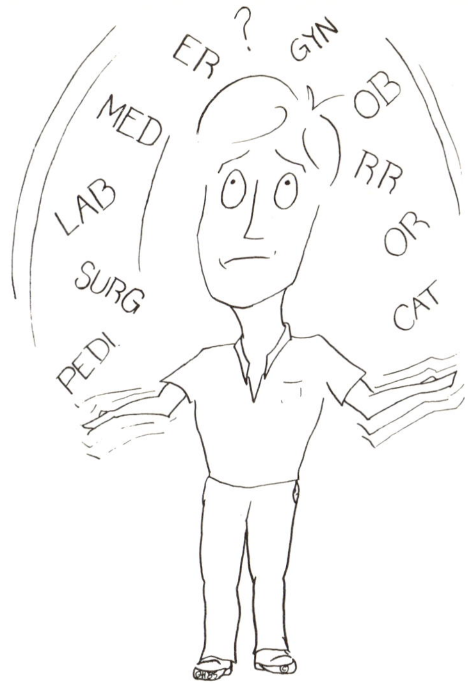

Figure 2.1 Initials and acronyms can be overwhelming in a hospital. (© Glen D. Hawkins).

intensive care unit and some have only the first two and care for cardiac patients in the medical unit.

The design of these units can vary, but generally all patients are electronically monitored and sometimes visible by video to the nurses' station. At no time is a patient left alone; he/ she is always under surveillance by the medical and nursing staffs. In hospitals with no medical house staff, the 24-hour responsibility is that of the nurses. When there are residents, interns, and medical students, some of these persons may also be present in the intensive care unit frequently, if not all the time.

There are restrictions on visitors in intensive care units. Only members of the immediate family and/or significant others can visit, and usually for a limited period of time every hour.

The length of time a patient remains in an intensive care unit varies, but discharge to a medical or surgical floor is usual once intensive monitoring and surveillance are no longer necessary. For most patients, discharge to a regular unit is a milestone and viewed as a turning point in their recovery.

Other specialty areas in the hospital include the obstetrical and the pediatric units. Not all hospitals have either of these. They are more likely to exist in hospitals in communities where the health care facilities are limited and the distance to another hospital is great.

The *obstetrical unit* includes the labor and delivery rooms, postpartum unit, the newborn nursery, and sometimes a special care or neonatal intensive care nursery. Should a hospital not have an intensive care nursery, infants requiring intensive care would be cared for in the newborn nursery and transferred to a children's hospital or to a regional center providing this care. Hospitals that provide only obstetrical and gynecological services have neonatal intensive care nurseries and generally serve as regional centers for this care. They also generally have facilities for prenatal inpatient care for women with high-risk pregnancies and special care for the postpartum care of women whose needs exceed normal care. Regionalization of neonatal care is well developed in this country. There are three levels of care: tertiary care, meaning a neonatal intensive care unit; secondary care, meaning a special care nursery, but without all the equipment and staff, for very intensive care of extremely sick or high-risk newborns; and routine newborn or level one care.

Some hospitals have *birthing rooms* in addition to the labor and delivery rooms. These rooms are more homelike spaces within the unit where women and their families can be together for both labor and delivery. For many persons, this is a compromise between 1) the more sterile and operating room atmosphere of a delivery room and 2) a home birth. The advantage of the birthing room over a home birth is that if a complication arises, the patient is in the hospital setting equipped to provide any emergency treatment or care.

The labor rooms are much like any hospital room and are usually private or semiprivate (two beds), or may even have three or four beds. The woman remains in the labor room until the delivery is imminent. The delivery rooms resemble operating rooms, sterile looking spaces where, if need be, a cesarean section could be performed. Once the woman has delivered and she and her baby have received their immediate post-delivery care, the baby is usually transferred to the newborn nursery and the woman to her room in the post-partum unit.

Many hospitals provide for mothers and babies to be together during their stay. This is called *rooming-in*. Mothers begin to care for their babies within a matter of hours after birth and the baby remains in the mother's room until discharge. The length of time mother and baby remain in the hospital can vary from 1 to 2 days postpartum to 7 to 10 days if the delivery was by cesarean section.

Pediatric units can also include adolescent care facilities. Most patients cared for in the pediatric units are those under sixteen. Hospitals with pediatric units often provide for mothers to remain with their children. This may be in the form of a cot for sleeping at night so the child is not alone. Children with serious illnesses are usually cared for in specialty children's hospitals so that most community hospital pediatric care is of a less serious nature and often for a shorter period of time

Some hospitals provide *orthopedic specialty areas.* These areas care for all patients with any orthopedic diagnoses.

Most of the beds are designed for trapeze connections, making it easier for patients to move themselves. A great number of these patients have had surgical hip replacement and are elderly patients with specialized needs. Should a hospital not have an orthopedic unit, these patients will be cared for in either the medical or surgical units, depending on their diagnoses.

Many hospitals, especially community hospitals, are including psychiatric units for short-term care. These are usually operated in conjunction with an outpatient psychotherapy program for followup care.

Some hospitals are providing specialty areas for the comprehensive treatment of *alcoholism.* These units provide detoxification services and therapy and include outpatient therapy after discharge.

A number of subspecialties exist within the practice of surgery and medicine. In large institutions, it is not uncommon to have patient care units devoted to these specialties; for example; neurology; neurosurgery; ear, eye, nose, and throat care (EENT); urology; gynecology; gastroenterology; thoracic care; plastic surgery; oncology; and so on. In smaller institutions, as we discussed earlier in this chapter, medical units and surgical units will have patients from some of these specialty areas.

Long-Term Services

Some hospitals offer patients long-term as well as acute care. In addition, there are hospitals offering only long-term care. These facilities are referred to as extended care or chronic care facilities. These services are often separate from the acute care hospital setting, but are part of the hospital complex. Veterans Administration hospitals often have long-term as well as short-term acute care patients. Of course, other hospitals can offer long-term care as well.

Much of the long-term care is rehabilitative in nature and is the result of the increase in the number of older adults with functional impairments that necessitate long-term care and skilled nursing care. Sometimes these patients are referred to nursing homes or extended care facilities that are separate entities when the hospital is no longer able to provide the long-term care that is needed and when the hospital has no special services to offer that the nursing home is unable to provide.

BY PRINCIPAL ORIENTATION

Hospitals may also be examined by their principal focus or mission. For purposes of our discussion, mission will be divided into community service, teaching, and commercial enterprise. Once again, as with virtually all the categories used throughout this book, these are not mutually exclusive classifications. A community hospital may have as a secondary mission teaching or a proprietary institution may affiliate with a medical or nursing school. From an idealistic perspective, perhaps all hospitals might be thought of as having community service as their first mission. In reality, although service to patients should be the primary mission of a hospital, sometimes that ideal is subsumed under other purposes.

Community Service

Community hospitals, operated on a nonprofit basis, perhaps come close to the ideal. They were usually built by the community, for the community, in order to provide hospital care for its residents when that becomes necessary. In fact, due to the changing character of communities, some community hospitals do not serve the community in which they are located, but serve another population residing at some distance from the institution. An example would be a community hospital unable to offer free services to a population dependent upon such services and without any other means to pay. Examples exist in many of our large cities. Often people have to travel across the city to the municipal or county hospital, rather than receive services from the non-profit community hospital down the block.

Teaching and Research

Teaching hospitals are either operated by or affiliated with schools of medicine, nursing, and other health professions. Their primary mission—teaching—is generally reflected in the patient population. Coupled closely with teaching and almost inherent in it is *clinical research*. Individuals with interesting or unusual conditions may be sought so that the students have the opportunity to learn. Patients using these hospitals are expected to be subjects for students and to be examined, questioned, and treated by many individuals. In recent years, attention to the rights of patients has helped to alter the "guinea pig" atmosphere, and health care providers have become much more sensitive to the dignity of the patient as a human being. It is important, of course, that patients in teaching hospitals understand the roles of the many persons whom they will meet during a hospital stay. Teaching hospitals offer patients the opportunity for care by teachers and their students, who must be up-to-date in the care they give and are often involved in research. People sometimes *choose* to be treated in teaching hospitals, feeling that the care will be superior to that offered in hospitals where the health care professionals are not stimulated to learn themselves by the questions of students.

The clinical center of the National Institutes for Health is perhaps the ultimate example of an institution devoted to research and, of course, teaching is part of the research process. Patients are referred and selected because their conditions are currently under investigation. They are offered the opportunity to be on the cutting edge of new treatments and are offered therapies perhaps available nowhere else in the world.

Commercial Enterprise

Hospitals run as commercial enterprises are becoming more numerous, as mentioned earlier in this chapter. Arguments are strong both for and against this kind of institution. Of course, they purport to have as their primary mission the care of patients, but that care will not continue over time if the business is unsuccessful. Perhaps, on the other hand, these institutions will demonstrate that quality care can be delivered in the context of a health care business for-profit and be cost-effective and satisfactory to patients.

REFERENCES

Statistical abstract of the United States, 1984 (1984). Washington, D.C.: U.S. Department of Commerce, Bureau of the Census.

Wilson, F.A. & Neuhauser, D. (1982). *Health services in the United States.* Cambridge, Mass.: Ballinger

3
Services Offered in Hospitals

The number and variety of services offered in any one hospital will depend upon: 1) the size of the institution, 2) the community to be served, 3) the needs of the population comprising that community, 4) sources of support for the hospital, 5) the availability of trained personnel to provide services, 6) the physical facilities and equipment the hospital possesses, and 7) the mission of the institution. For example, a small community hospital in a relatively rural area with an aging target population, two family practice physicians, one surgeon, and the closest school of nursing 100 miles away would need to provide very different services than a large urban medical center affiliated with several schools educating health care professionals that receives referral patients from all over the geographic region. A hospital located in a suburb of a large metropolitan area would also need to consider what services it could best provide and what equipment to purchase, taking into account when it would be best to refer patients to specialists at a medical center. In the last chapter, we discussed the speciality services that a hospital might offer to its patients. In this chapter, we will discuss diagnostic and therapeutic services and then describe typical inpatient residential care in a hospital.

DIAGNOSTIC SERVICES

The diagnostic services of a hospital are an essential aspect of the medical care of the community. They are also becoming big business for hospitals and involve the expenditure of large amounts of money for equipment. These services are utilized on both an inpatient and outpatient basis. Some larger hospitals have the capability of providing all the diagnostic services that have been developed, from the simplest laboratory urine test to the most complex process utilizing computers and huge scanning machines. Other hospitals can only provide the more commonly needed and used services. For example, all hospitals have x-ray departments and laboratories capable of providing basic diagnostic information when needed. Some larger hospitals or groups of hospitals may share more expensive diagnostic services and equipment such as the computerized axial tomography (CAT) scanner. With ever rising costs and the need for cost containment, sharing of resources and personnel rather than duplication is becoming more necessary in the diagnostic services hospitals provide.

Because of the high cost of exploratory surgery to the patient physically, emotionally, and financially, more emphasis than ever before is being placed on accurate diagnosis. Technology has responded through research being conducted to make available newer, less invasive, and more cost-effective methods to aid in the diagnosis of disease.

In the sections to follow, we will discuss diagnostic services more fully to provide you with some understanding of the types of services a hospital can provide. As a nurse, you will prepare patients for diagnostic procedures and teach them what to expect.

Common Laboratory Tests

We have not attempted to describe every possible test here, nor have we even attempted to describe all of those that are most common. We have chosen examples to indicate to you the variety of tests available. Many fine references to common laboratory tests are available. Some of these are listed in the bibliography at the end of the book for your convenience.

The *complete blood count* (CBC) is such a common test that virtually all of us will have it done several times. This test is almost always done when a person has a complete health assessment and physical examination in order to provide a total picture of that individual's health. The complete blood count includes a hematocrit (the volume percentage of erythrocytes in whole blood), hemoglobin (the oxygen-carrying pigment of the erythrocytes, formed by the developing erythrocyte in bone marrow), leukocyte or white blood cell count, and an erythrocyte or red blood cell count.

The FBS or *fasting blood sugar* detects the presence of glucose in the blood and, as the name implies, is done after the patient has fasted for a specified period of time. It is useful in screening for and diagnosis of diabetes, as well as other conditions.

The *glucose tolerance test* (GTT) is a test that is usually ordered on an individual when the presence of diabetes is suspected. It is more specific than the fasting blood sugar. All patients with a family history of diabetes who are concerned about this condition should avail themselves of the fasting blood sugar test and/or this test.

The BUN *(blood urea nitrogen)* is one of the tests of kidney function. As the name implies, it is a blood test.

Probably most of you have heard of measuring cholesterol. *Cholesterol level* is one index of risk for heart attack. More persons are having this test done because of the high incidence of cardiovascular conditions among the adult population in this country. It is a useful test to discover if one's diet may be too high in saturated fats and points to the need for altering one's diet and lifestyle to lower the risk of cardiovascular diseases, including heart attack, high blood pressure, and stroke. Tests can also be conducted to measure levels of other fats in the blood (triglycerides, high density lipids) to give a profile of cardiovascular risk.

The *urinalysis* is as common as the complete blood count, a test that each of us probably has had many times. It is sometimes referred to as UA. It is an analysis of the urine for infection (presence of bacteria), as well as glucose, protein, red and white blood cells, pus, ph, and specific gravity.

A urine culture can also be done to determine which organisms and how many are present in the urine. A *culture and sensitivity* (C & S) is done to determine the offending organism and which antibiotic or sulfa drug will be most effective in combatting the infection [which one(s) the organism is sensitive to]. This test is also useful in general screening for diabetes (presence of glucose) and kidney disorders (bacteria, pus, protein, specific gravity), but it is not specific for these conditions, and further studies would need to be done.

With the current concern about cancer of the bowel, the *guaiac test* is becoming routine to uncover hidden blood in the stool. This may also be referred to as a test for occult blood. Any time there is a suspicion that the person is bleeding anywhere in the gastrointestinal tract, this test should be done. It is a reliable, inexpensive test that can be done by anyone, and has proven to be an excellent tool in the early detection of many conditions, including cancer of the colon.

When a person is suspected of having tuberculosis, one of the tests that can be done is the AFB *(acid fast bacillus)*. This test is done on sputum. Throat cultures are swabs of the throat and tonsillar areas to diagnose the presence of bacterial infection, especially streptococcus. Of course, cultures can be done of virtually any part of the body and of body wastes and secretions, such as urine, stool, vaginal, and breast discharges, of a skin lesion, mucous membrane, wound, or surgical site.

Laboratory tests also include examination of cells and organs or tissues, known as 1) cytology or 2) cytopathology and pathology. A common example is the examination of cells scraped from the surface of the cervix, known as the Pap (Papanicolaou for its developer) smear or Pap test. This test for cancer of the cervix can detect early changes in cervical cells even before cancer is present. Another example is the study of cells obtained by amniocentesis from the fetal sac during a pregnancy. A genetic study of cells is also possible; the study of the genetic makeup of cells is a separate specialty, sometimes referred to in the generic as genetics. The study of cells can also be done from the fluid obtained with a gastric lavage (fluid inserted and then removed or aspirated).

When tissue is removed, whether it be a mole; skin tab; a polyp from the bowel, nose, cervix, or other site; or part or all of an organ, such as the lung, uterus, stomach, and so on, the tissue must be examined for the presence or absence of disease. Tissue means a clump of cells, be it only a few cells, a section, or an entire organ or foreign mass. The most complete examination of all organs can occur only when a person has died. This is known as an autopsy and virtually all hospital laboratories have a special area for conducting autopsies and storing bodies until they are released for burial. Autopsies are done to investigate or confirm cause of death. They are also useful for research into the detection, treatment, and cure of disease.

It is obvious from this brief discussion that the scope of services the hospital laboratory can offer is very wide. Typically, in the laboratory we can analyze all body secretions, all excretions, and all organs and tissues both normal and foreign, be the latter benign or malignant. A particular laboratory may not have the personnel or equipment necessary to do very specialized tests, certain cultures of bacteria or viruses, or highly specialized tissue and organ analyses. Referral to larger hospital laboratories, to state health department laboratory facilities, or to the laboratories of the Centers for Disease Control in Atlanta, Georgia, or the National Institutes for Health Clinical Center in Bethesda, Maryland, both part of the U.S. Public Health Service, Department of Health and Human Services, is possible.

Diagnostic Technology

With the advent of newer and more complex equipment to aid in the diagnosing of disease, hospitals have had to make available a broader range of services to patients. One major advantage of new technology is that many of these services can be utilized on an outpatient basis. Perhaps the area of radiology has received the lion's share of diagnostic capabilities utilized on an outpatient basis. These studies can include the more conventional x-rays of the chest, upper and lower gastrointestinal tract (barium swallow and barium enema), those used to rule out fractures of almost every bone in the body, and the more sophisticated methods such as ultrasound, the CAT scan, and mammography. In the next section, we will attempt to outline and discuss briefly some of the diagnostic tools and services available today.

The *CAT scanner,* or CAT scan as it has become known, is the darling of modern health care technology. Within seconds, the sophisticated imagery system of a full body scanner can be used to diagnose accurately. This marvelous tool can be used to detect a myriad of conditions—from cerebral hemorrhages and tumors to lower back problems. This broad range makes the CAT scanner a miraculous invention, an important adjunct to conventional x-ray techniques, and an indispensable diagnostic tool. The correct term for the CAT scanner is computerized axial tomography. What this machine does is to produce cross-sectional photographic images of the body by combining x-ray and computer technology.

How simple it is for a person to lie on a sliding table that is moving slowly through the hollow opening at one end of the machine while invisible x-ray beams are making readings. As the table moves slowly, it stops to take pictures along the way. The whole process takes anywhere from three-quarters to 1 hour to complete.

One thing that can be frightening to patients having a CAT scan, however, is that during the procedure whirling sounds can be heard that are a normal part of the machine's operation. Some specialized head scans will require an injection of dye for contrast images and visualization of cranial structures, but otherwise it is a noninvasive procedure. The capabilities of the CAT scan have reduced the need for other more painful and invasive procedures. There is little risk to patients and it is considerably less time-consuming than previously used diagnostic tests.

Ultrasound is also referred to as sonogram and is a painless, noninvasive procedure employing the use of sonar (sound) waves at very high speed (thus the "ultra") to visualize and trace organs in the body, as well as to visualize the gestational sac, the uterus, and the fetus in the pregnant woman. The principle of ultrasound is the use of high frequency sound waves to trace the particular pattern of an organ or area of the body, such as the pregnant uterus. The procedure can vary slightly, depending upon the part of the body being traced. For example, if the abdominal or pelvic cavity is being addressed, the patient lies in a supine position and the technician, using a wand, will rub it over the area to be examined. Mineral oil is applied to the area to facilitate maximum contact between the skin and the wand, also allowing the wand to glide easily and smoothly over the skin's surface. An image or picture is produced on a screen much like a television screen, and photographs may be taken of the images if and when these are needed. Any time the abdominal or pelvic area is being scanned, the patient is instructed to have a full bladder, because it is used as an anatomical landmark.

Ultrasound is especially valuable in obstetrics. The presence of the gestational sac can confirm pregnancy. The age and position of the fetus, the diagnosing of multiple pregnancy, and the differential diagnosis of placenta previa (low lying placenta) have made the ultrasound technique widely used in clinical practice. Ultrasound is also used to detect fetal heartbeat. Small, hand-held ultrasound devices can be used in place of traditional fetoscopes.

Another use of ultrasound is in what is called *echo cardiography* or the echo cardiogram. Here, the procedure is somewhat altered, but the principle is the same. Sonar waves are used to trace the pattern and function of the heart. The procedure differs in that three electrical leads, like those used in an electrocardiogram, are attached to the chest for monitoring the heartbeat and then a small probe or transducer is surfaced over the left chest area. This will allow the sonar waves to beam in different directions in order to visualize the entire heart, valves, chambers, and muscle, as the heart beats. This painless procedure takes less than an hour.

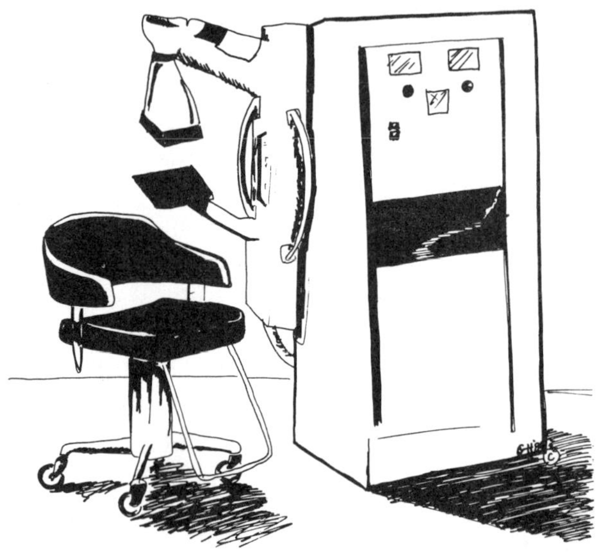

Figure 3.1 Mammography Machine. (© Glen D. Hawkins).

Mammography is another diagnostic service offered by some hospitals for detection of breast cancer. It is a special technique for x-raying the breasts. With the incidence of breast cancer so high, and the number 2 cause of death in adult women, there is considerable justification for providing this diagnostic service in most hospitals. It is an accurate, painless, noninvasive outpatient procedure that can reduce the dreaded fear of breast cancer among women and greatly assist the physician in making a diagnosis. A mammogram can eliminate needless biopsies and reduce the patient's anxiety almost immediately. If cancer is detected, the survival rate increases significantly if it is diagnosed in its very earliest stages. In women over the age of 35, and some say 40, many health care providers include mammography as part of the routine health examination, if there is a family history of breast cancer (mother, sister). For women without a family history or other high risk factors, a baseline mammogram may be done when the woman is 45 or 50 and thereafter every 2 to 3 years. Protocols vary depending upon many factors, including the woman's history and any previous breast conditions, as well as risk for developing breast cancer.

The radiation dose used in mammography is very low and considered within the range of minimal risk, especially in the context of the risk of developing breast cancer. One breast is examined at a time. The breast being examined is placed on a sill, with the patient sitting facing the machine, and the breast will be compressed slightly between the x-ray tube and the film. This compression is an important aspect of the mammogram. The entire procedure with two or more x-rays taken, requires no special preparation beforehand and takes less than an hour to complete.

Under the umbrella of *nuclear medicine* come all the tests involving the use of radioactive isotopes. The tests done using this nuclear material are varied and several will be discussed here.

The lung scan involves an evaluation of the blood supply to the lungs and how air passes in and out. The first of these is called a perfusion scan and the latter, a ventilation scan. To evaluate the blood supply, a dye is injected into the veins to provide contrast, and photographs are taken from various angles using a gamma camera. To examine how air passes in and out of the lungs, breathing through a mouthpiece or face mask is required. A small amount of radioactive gas will be added to oxygen in the tubing and the patient will be asked to breathe normally, maintaining a tight seal around the device, while photographs are taken. Both procedures are safe, painless, and take less than an hour to complete.

For a brain scan, a radioactive dye is injected into the vein and photographs are taken using the gamma camera as the dye travels to the brain via the blood.

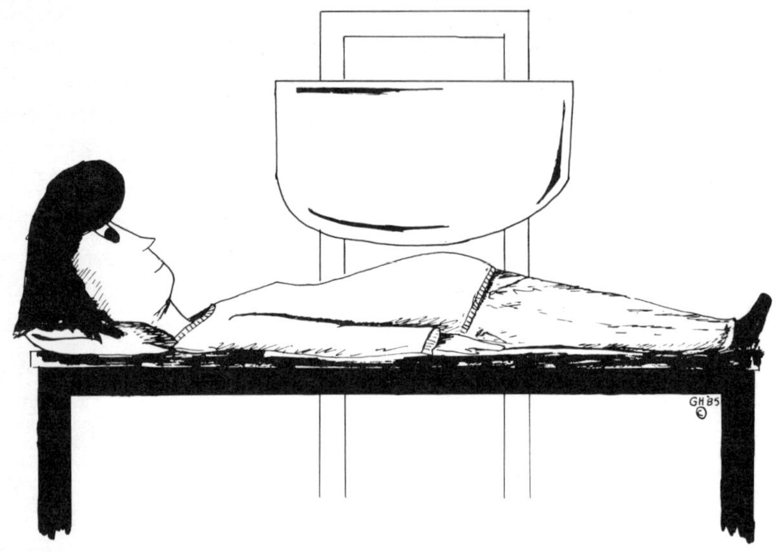

Figure 3.2 Gamma Camera. (© Glen D. Hawkins).

The same dye is used for bone scans. It is injected and then pictures are taken of the bones. This scan takes longer than a brain scan, as the photographs cannot be taken until the bones have received the radioactive dye. The process can take more than 2 to 3 hours after injection of the material. The patient is instructed to drink plenty of fluids and to void frequently, so that the dye not collected in the bones will pass out through the urine. Once the bones have received the dye, full body photographs are taken.

Scans of the liver and spleen are possible through a very similar technique. A radioactive dye is injected and photographs are taken to see the blood flowing from the arteries and veins into the liver. Other photographs in different directions can be taken as well, including the spleen.

Renal scans make possible examination of the urinary system and photographs of the kidneys. Again radioactive dye is used and photographs are taken.

A thyroid uptake and scan is yet another test utilizing radioactive material. These tests examine the thyroid gland and involve a preparation time of 1 day. The patient swallows a capsule containing radioactive iodine and 24 hours later, a probe is placed over the neck to measure the amount of the radioactive iodine substance in the thyroid gland to determine its functioning. For the scan, radioactive isotopes are injected into a vein and photographs are taken 20 minutes later, once the material has collected in the thyroid gland.

The thallium-201 stress exam is a stress test, quite vigorous in nature, that evaluates the adequacy of the blood supply to the heart muscle using radioactive isotopes. Thallium-201 is injected intravenously during peak exercise. Several leads are attached to the patient's chest and connected to an electrocardiograph machine to monitor heart rhythm. The exercises used in the stress test can be 1) the treadmill, or

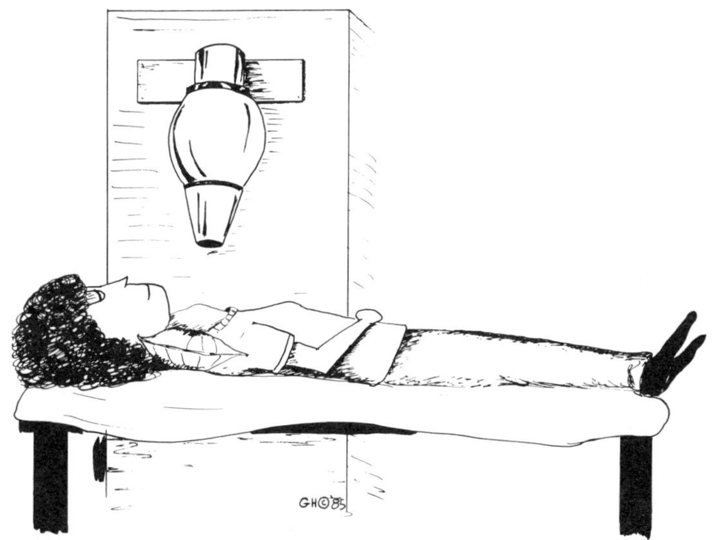

Figure 3.3 Machine for doing thyroid uptake and scan. (© Glen D. Hawkins).

2) the stationary bicycle, or 3) both. The pace begins slowly, increasing to a peak. The radioactive isotope will be injected into a venous line about 1 minute before the end of the exercise session. Immediately after the exercise portion of the exam, photographs are taken at different angles with the camera held very close to the chest and the patient lying flat on his/her back.

Preparation for this test may involve withholding certain cardiac medication prescribed for the patient, but that decision is left to the patient's physician. Usually the suggestion is made that the patient refrain from food or drink for several hours before the test to avoid the possibility of nausea during the strenuous exercise session.

Special Diagnostic X-ray Examinations

X-ray is one of the oldest and most common of the "modern" technological diagnostic tools. Conventional x-ray is used for detection of changes that are dense enough to impede the passage of x-rays, such as the calcifications caused by tuberculosis of the lungs and dense tumors of the organs or bones. Since bones are made of dense material, injury or anomaly can generally be detected on x-ray, such as a fracture or areas where calcium has been lost. Special x-ray techniques have also been developed using materials that enhance visibility of a condition or organ, and these are discussed later in this chapter.

An *intravenous pyelogram* (IVP) is an x-ray of the urinary tract. A contrast dye is injected into the veins and allowed to circulate into the urinary system. X-rays are taken and, when developed, any abnormalities can be seen readily.

Upper and lower gastrointestinal series, also known as an upper g.i. and a lower g.i., and sometimes including a *gall bladder series* as well, are common diagnostic procedures that have been possible for many years to diagnose abnormalities within the gastrointestinal tract and the gall bladder. These are now supplemented, of course, by newer techniques such as scope exams.

The preparation is simple. For the upper gastrointestinal series, no special preparation is necessary. For the lower series, laxatives and the small enema used for the sigmoidoscopy are done by the patient at home the day or evening before. If a gall bladder series is included, teleopaque tablets which contain an opaque dye are swallowed at intervals of a few minutes until all are gone. A light, fat free diet is advised the evening before the x-ray and nothing per os (NPO) that is, nothing by mouth, after midnight.

The procedure is as follows: for the upper gastrointestinal series, a milkshake of barium is swallowed by the patient to better visualize the digestive tract on x-ray. Sometimes fluoroscopy is used during the procedure to view the swallowing mechanism and observe the barium passing into the stomach and small intestine. For the lower gastrointestinal series, a barium enema is given by the x-ray technician for the same purpose, to contrast the bowel on x-ray. A series of x-rays is taken and the patient is encouraged to expel the barium once the procedure is over. A mild laxative may be given to assist the person in expelling all the barium from the bowel. For the gall bladder series, x-rays are taken because the contrast dye provided by the teleopaque tablets swallowed the evening before provide for complete visualization.

The patient can eat or drink once the x-rays are taken and resume normal activities. Patients should be told that their stools may be white from the barium for the first day or so after the test.

Chest x-ray is probably so common that nearly all of us have had one at one time or another. A chest x-ray is sometimes required as part of a pre-employment health examination, especially for health care providers. This x-ray allows for direct visualization of the heart and lungs. It is an excellent screening tool for conditions such as bronchitis, tuberculosis, pneumonia, and other lung diseases. It can also detect such conditions as an enlarged heart. It is used routinely on nearly all hospital admissions (unless one has just been done on a particular patient) and on anyone undergoing day surgery.

Noninvasive Tests

A few hospitals have begun to include diagnostic laboratories that aid in the discovery of problems in the vascular system. The equipment used in diagnosing vascular problems and abnormalities is painless, reliable, and risk-free, but best of all, it is noninvasive. All the tests in this category can be done on an outpatient basis. To give an example of how much time and money is saved with this service, we will use the case of a patient suspected of having phlebitis, an inflammation of a vein or veins, or a deep vein thrombosis (clot in a vein) that can be life-threatening. Without the laboratory capacity for doing these noninvasive tests, this patient would be hospitalized, on complete bedrest, and given anticoagulant therapy to reduce the risk of clot formation. Doppler ultrasound is one of these noninvasive methods and works on the same principle as other ultrasonic devices, utilizing sound waves to detect changes in density in the extremity. Another noninvasive method of detecting a venous problem is impedance plethysmography, utilization of a device to measure and record changes in volume in venous return from the limb in which the clot or phlebitis is suspected. With the noninvasive vascular tests now available, within 30 minutes, a definitive diagnosis can be made or the condition ruled out and the patient free to go about life as usual.

Electrocardiogram (EKG) is a common diagnostic tool. It is widely used in physicians' offices, clinics, and hospitals. It is a painless, noninvasive procedure with no special preparation necessary. The public has become so familiar with this tool that patients frequently need little or no explanation about the procedure. The EKG measures the electrical activity of the heart to see if the rate and rhythm are within a normal range and limit. Electrodes are applied to the chest and extremities and recordings are made on a narrow strip of printout paper. There are now also portable units about the size of a micro tape recorder that a person can wear going about daily activities. A recording is made of the reading and then can be interpreted by a physician.

Electroencephalogram (EEG) is the companion examination to the EKG. This diagnostic tool measures brain activity and is a painless procedure using electrodes attached to areas of the head. The readout is similar to that of the EKG. The electrical activity of the brain is being recorded, sometimes referred to as the brain waves. Sometimes a person will be asked to wear a portable unit to record during normal activities or to have a recording going all night to examine nocturnal activity.

Examinations Using a Lighted Scope

Endoscopy is an invasive procedure that can be done on an outpatient basis to diagnose, biopsy, and in some instances treat inaccessible parts of the body. Prior to endoscopy, some areas such as the stomach were impossible to view without exploratory surgery or the crude method of outlining with a contrast medium like barium. The development of fiber optics, the same technology now being used in telephone communications and many other fields, has made possible the development of flexible lighted scopes with incredibly small diameters. With the advent of endoscopy, looking from within, a whole new focus of diagnosing and treating came into being. Never before had one been able to rule out a diagnosis such as gastric ulcers in an outpatient setting with such confidence, and with minimal discomfort to the patient.

In this procedure, a flexible tube or rod is inserted through the mouth into the area of the gastrointestinal tract to be examined. A lighted tube and probe may also be passed within the outer tube for better visualization of the area and possible biopsy. The biopsy capability can aid greatly in differential diagnoses and determine any malignancy.

The preparation for endoscopy is very simple. The patient can have no food or drink from midnight of the previous day. This prevents the possibility of vomiting and aspiration. The person is given some mild sedation or tranquilizer drug and the throat is sprayed with an anesthetic to reduce the gag reflex. After this minimal preparation and explanation to the patient of what to expect, the endoscope is passed by the examiner and the procedure completed. The length of time necessary varies, depending on whether biopsies are taken or if any treatment, such as cauterization of a blood vessel, is attempted or carried out.

Once the endoscope is removed, the patient may experience some swelling and irritation of the throat; this discomfort is understandable. An ice pack on the neck and frequent observation of the patient until swelling is reduced are advisable. Food or drink is usually withheld until the swallow and gag reflexes are back to normal. Once the patient can swallow comfortably and throat swelling is substantially reduced, the patient can be allowed to go home. Eating and drinking should be avoided for several hours, and once all reflexes are normal, liquids should be encouraged. Endoscopy has saved thousands of dollars in medical and hospital fees, loss of employment, needless surgery, and overall trauma to patients.

Bronchoscopy is also an invasive procedure that allows for direct visualization of the bronchial tubes and trachea. The preparation of the patient is the same as for endoscopy; however, the procedure is slightly different. The patient is placed lying flat on his/her back with the head dropped back slightly off the table but supported. This allows for the best alignment and easiest passage of the bronchoscope. The instrument used is rigid rather than flexible, but has the same openings for light and probe. The possibilities for biopsy and treatment are the same as with endoscopy.

The recuperation of the patient is much the same, except that it may take longer for the throat swelling to go down because the scope passed is rigid and the possibility of tissue trauma is present. Observation of the patient, an ice collar to the neck, and withholding of anything by mouth will assure complete recovery in a matter of hours.

Sigmoidoscopy is an invasive procedure allowing for direct visualization of the lower gastrointestinal tract up to the sigmoid portion of the colon—hence the name. This examination used to be done with a long rigid scope, but newer advances have made possible a more flexible tube that gives only minimal discomfort to the patient. This has been reduced to an office procedure and is often done annually for any patients with bowel conditions.

The preparation is done by the patient at home the day before the scheduled exam. It usually involves laxatives and small, concentrated, disposable unit enemas (that have come to be known by the trade name under which they were first marketed, Fleet ®) to insure that the intestine is empty and clear for visualization. A light diet is encouraged beforehand to reduce bowel activity until after the procedure. The exam takes only about 15 minutes with minimal discomfort, a pressure-like feeling experienced by the patient. Biopsies and treatment can be performed during the procedure. Once the exam is over, the patient may go about his/her daily activities, including eating and drinking, immediately.

Colonoscopy is yet another invasive procedure that allows for direct visualization of the entire large intestine. This procedure requires more preparation than with other exams. Besides laxatives, the patient will have several enemas, usually large soapsud enemas, until the return is clear. The "bowel prep," as this is called, is necessary to be sure that the entire colon can be visualized. The patient is usually given a sedative before this procedure, as there is likely to be a moderate degree of discomfort. The flexible colonoscope is inserted into the rectum and allowed to pass through the entire length of the large bowel, visualizing and taking biopsies whenever needed. The entire procedure can last an hour, depending upon what is done. After the colonoscopy, the patient is observed for signs of bleeding and/or abdominal pain. Food and drink may be given soon after the patient is alert, as the effects of the sedative wear off.

A *cystoscopy* is a diagnostic tool for looking directly into the bladder. It is an "invasive procedure" because a rigid instrument is passed through the urethra into the bladder. Biopsies and treatment can be undertaken during the exam. This is a relatively short procedure with little or no preparation needed beforehand.

A *laparoscopy* is a more invasive procedure requiring anesthesia in order to insert a lighted scope into the lower abdominal cavity to examine the contents, including uterus, tubes, and ovaries. The preparation of the patient is similar to that for minor surgical procedures involving general anesthesia; nothing to eat or drink after midnight the evening before, chest x-ray, blood work, and sometimes an electrocardiogram the day before the surgery (or it could be 2 or more days before), and sometimes shaving of the abdomen from breasts to pubic area. After the patient is asleep, a small incision is made in the umbilical area and another in the right lower quadrant. The lighted scope (laparoscope) is inserted into the former incision, and a probe to guide the scope is inserted into the lower incision. Biopsies can be taken and a tubal ligation performed. This procedure can be done on a day surgery basis, with the patient coming in early in the morning, having the procedure done, recovering from the anesthesia, and going home the same day.

THERAPIES

Hospitals are in the business not only of diagnosing what is wrong with people but of trying to cure them. The generic term for the curing process is called therapy. Of course, not all therapy is curative. It may be restorative in nature, enabling an individual to live a better life despite a particular condition, such as orthopedic surgery to improve the gait of a person with cerebral palsy. It may be palliative, enabling the person to have less discomfort during the part of life remaining, such as the severing of a nerve tract to relieve chronic pain in a person with terminal cancer. Nonetheless, medical science always strives to find more cures for diseases that at present are beyond our grasp and to improve therapeutic techniques for those conditions for which there may never be a cure, but for which significant improvement may be possible. Hospitals are not the only sites for treatment and curing of disease, of course. Most health care takes place in the community, but hospitals offer the advantages of specialized equipment and highly educated health care professionals to provide care and, when possible, cure. In addition, much research is conducted in hospitals, especially those affiliated with medical schools and other professional schools, including nursing. Without research, there would be few advancements in the quest for effective treatments and cures for disease. In this section, we will discuss the common therapies that a hospital can offer its patients.

Curative

Surgery is the curative therapy that comes to mind perhaps first and foremost. This may be because of the frequency with which it is performed and the fact that for so many years, it was the singular form of treatment for a wide variety of maladies. Interestingly, surgery is also virtually as old as humankind, although of course ancient attempts were rarely successful. The 19th century developments of anesthesia and sepsis made possible surgery that could offer a reasonable chance of recovery. Today, the pendulum is beginning to swing in another direction, with surgery being viewed as simply one form of treatment available among many for conditions previously treated only by removal or at least alteration of the offending tissue or organ. Surgery will still occupy its place as an important remedy for many health problems, however, and will probably remain the therapy of choice for a significant set of conditions that no other curative or therapeutic interventions can match. The typical hospital has hundreds of cases of surgery a year, ranging from simple, short procedures done under local anesthesia, often done as day surgery, to extensive, invasive, long cases for rebuilding, removal, or even replacement of one or more organs. Many hospitals now offer surgery both on a day surgery basis (come in that morning and go home the same day) and for inpatients who will require skilled nursing care before and after surgery from 24 hours to days or weeks of recuperation.

Chemotherapy is a form of treatment that has become a driving force with the advent of newer and more powerfully effective drugs that have become available for general use on cancer patients. Often as a curative therapy, chemotherapy or drug treatment is used in conjunction with other therapies, such as surgery. Chemotherapy can be used alone, however, and can be the treatment of choice for certain diseases. Leukemia is an example of a disease that responds most effectively to chemotherapy. Chemotherapy by its name implies the administration of certain drugs, known as chemotherapeutics, to effect treatment or cure.

Needless to say, these drugs can have numerous side effects which can often elicit the response that the treatment is worse than the disease. This is not true, of course, but it demonstrates clearly the severity of side effects that can be experienced by those receiving chemotherapy. As health care providers, we should never let this fact escape our consciousness and should do all that we can to be supportive and therapeutic when caring for these patients.

Nausea and vomiting are very common side effects of chemotherapeutics and the degree to which an individual can experience these symptoms can vary from mild to severe. Treating the symptoms to alleviate as much discomfort as possible is in order for all patients receiving these drugs.

Patients receiving this form of therapy may be hospitalized for several days a month while receiving chemotherapy or may receive it on an outpatient basis. The drugs are administered both by mouth and by intravenous route. Some patients receive more than one drug and will have schedules for each that may differ, as will the route of administration. Some hospitals with many patients receiving chemotherapy will have a special unit for these persons to receive their therapy on either an ambulatory and/or an inpatient short-term basis. Often the nurses will come to know the patients and their families well over the course of their therapy and can be very helpful and supportive.

Radiation is another example of curative therapy that is widely used. It can be used alone or in conjunction with other therapies and can be the treatment of choice for certain malignancies. Once again, this therapy is not without some side effects, most notably alopecia or hair loss, and skin irritation at the radiation site, resembling a severe sunburn. This therapy is usually done on an outpatient basis.

Radium implantation is a curative therapy that is useful in certain specific cases where localization is possible or necessary. Tubules of radium are implanted into the affected area for a certain amount of time. Usually the patient is hospitalized when receiving this form of therapy, since it is radioactive. Health care professionals providing care generally wear badges that monitor the amount of radiation they are receiving to protect them from overexposure.

Laser therapy is a more recent addition to the curative therapeutic armament and is used very successfully in areas that are hard to reach or are inaccessible, such as the eye. Certain eye conditions, usually near the retina and often causing gradual loss of sight, can be corrected through the use of laser therapy. Laser treatment has been very useful in the treatment of diabetic retinopathy, a condition of the retina that is not uncommon in persons with diabetes and is a common cause of blindness. The laser seals the tiny vessels without an incision or anesthesia being required and with only minimal discomfort. Laser therapy is also being used for certain neurosurgery procedures that involve pinpointing an area in the brain. It is being used in gynecology to treat conditions of the cervix without surgery.

Laser therapy was developed in the 1960s, and produces high concentrations of light that can be focused minutely on an affected area. The beam can seal hemorrhages, relieve pressure within the eye (as in the case of glaucoma), and even re-attach retinas. It can destroy minute amounts of abnormal tissue without destroying the surrounding normal areas and is much more precise and less invasive than surgery.

Medications as cure deserve at least passing mention, as many, if not most, hospital patients receive medications. Some, such as antibiotics, may be used for curing disease. For the most part, however, persons are not hospitalized just to receive medications for cure of illness.

Rehabilitative Therapies

Physical therapy as a form of treatment seems to be growing at an accelerated rate. More and more health care professionals are realizing the advantages of early and sometimes vigorous physical therapy for patients with a wide range of conditions. This has been greeted by the consumer with positive acceptance. Perhaps the growing emphasis on physical fitness in this country and a host of other factors, including the desire to remain independent and take responsibility for self care, contribute to the positive attitude of consumers.

Patients who have suffered cerebral vascular accidents or strokes have been greatly aided by physical therapy as soon as their conditions have stabilized, often within days of the injury. Getting rehabilitation soon has decreased the effects of immobility and paralysis. Patients who have had total hip replacement or other joint replacement are up ambulating with walkers within a day or 2 after surgery. Because many of these persons are older adults, early physical activity has a positive effect on their overall well-being and recovery.

Victims of sports related injuries, vehicular accident victims, and a host of other conditions, some related to disease, too numerous to mention also have profited in recovery time or extent of recovery from this therapy.

Physical therapy has many aspects besides exercise and walking. Whirlpool therapy, massage, crutch walking, exercises for selected joints, such as the shoulders, and progressive weight bearing are examples. Most hospitals offer physical therapy both on an inpatient and an outpatient basis. Physical therapists will visit patients who are hospitalized in their rooms and begin therapy or the patient can be transported to the physical therapy unit. Plans will be made for continuation of therapy after discharge as needed, either through referral to a community agency offering this service or through return of the patient to the hospital for continuation of therapy on an outpatient basis.

Respiratory therapy is common to many patients during a hospital stay. During a typical hospitalization, a large proportion of patients receive one form or another of this therapy. This demonstrates how widely used it is and the importance placed upon it. Patients undergoing surgery can be at risk for pneumonia postoperatively. Respiratory therapy has aided greatly in preventing this from happening. Patients, in addition to being encouraged to cough and deep breathe to loosen lung secretions, are taught, for example, to use blow bottles. This is a form of incentive spirometry. When the patient blows into the mouthpiece, ping-pong like balls are raised to a certain level or fluid is moved from one bottle to another if he/she is breathing deeply enough. Either type of setup assists the patient in deep breathing and provides positive visual feedback that he/she is voluntarily aiding and improving his/her own condition.

Chest percussion also assists in promoting drainage of pulmonary secretions and the use of intermittent positive pressure breathing (IPPB) devices that encourage hyperventilation of the lungs by applying positive pressure to the airways is another form of respiratory therapy. Oxygen administration generally comes under the rubric of respiratory therapy. Many patients in the hospital receive oxygen, either by nasal cannula or mask or tent, for a variety of conditions. The respiratory therapy department generally assumes responsibility for the setup, maintenance, and removal of all oxygen and other respiratory equipment, and also provides certain therapies to patients. Nurses, too, provide some forms of respiratory therapy, such as helping a patient to cough and deep breathe after surgery, teaching the techniques before surgery, and performance of chest percussion, as well as monitoring oxygen therapy and starting it up or discontinuing it, as the condition of the patient warrants. The respiratory therapist cannot be at the patient's bedside 24 hours a day, but nurses are.

Occupational therapy is a therapy that is being used more widely than ever before. Many patients are unaware of the occupational therapy department until they come to use its services.

Occupational therapists help patients to perform the simple activities of daily living that we all take for granted. Patients with disabilities, victims of strokes with or without paralysis, patients with spinal cord injuries, and those with amputations are among those who benefit from occupational therapy.

Very often these therapists work with other health care professionals to determine the best course of therapy for a client and how it should be implemented. It may be necessary for the occupational therapist to visit the patient's home to help determine how activities of daily living or the environment can best be modified to accommodate any long-term compromise of ability. The therapist also works with family members to help keep the patient as independent and actively involved in his or her own care and responsibilities as possible.

The woman who has had a radical or modified mastectomy (removal of the breast) for cancer is a good example. She will probably have difficulty raising the arm on the affected side. The *physical therapist* will teach and encourage range of motion or other arm exercises to promote return of full mobility or use of the arm, and the *occupational therapist* will instruct the patient in activities that encourage this mobility and show how to adapt normal activities to provide the needed exercise. This interdisciplinary approach to patient care is part of the emerging picture in health care.

Many of the activities used in occupational therapy are overlooked by many health care professionals, and it takes a practiced eye to recognize that a simple pleasurable activity like weaving can do wonders for a patient, physically and emotionally. Many of the activities of the occupational therapy department are aimed at restoration of full activity, as well as mental well-being; making the person feel useful; being able to resume caring for self and others; and engaging in activities that provide social activities and pass the time when long hospitalization is necessary.

Speech therapy is an area that is sometimes included in the interdisciplinary approach to rehabilitative care. If a patient has suffered a stroke, the care will include physical and occupational therapy and, if speech is affected because of the location of the cerebral insult, the person is also a candidate for speech therapy.

There are other conditions requiring this therapy alone, including patients who have had surgery for cancer of the larynx. Esophageal speech, the process of swallowing air to bring about sound and produce speech, can be taught by speech therapists. Any patient having corrective surgery for a cleft palate or other malformations or injuries affecting speech or the larynx can benefit from speech therapy.

Voice therapy, although usually offered on an outpatient basis, may be offered by a hospital to ambulatory clients. This is therapy to treat injuries, either physical or psychosocial, that affect one's voice, for example shouting or talking a great deal, resulting in alteration in the sound of one's voice. Singers, politicians, lawyers, and others whose voices are their profession benefit from voice therapy.

Palliative Therapy

Palliative therapies are those that are offered to patients when there is virtually no hope of a cure for the disease. These are designed to do just what the term suggests: to offer at least temporary relief from the effects of the disease process, to increase the patient's comfort and offer relief from pain, and, in some cases, to keep the person alive until a more permanent resolution can be attempted or is developed. An example of the latter is kidney dialysis that is used for some patients until a kidney transplant can be attempted. There are several examples of palliative therapy we will discuss, the first of which is dialysis.

Dialysis is a form of therapy for those persons with such severe difficulties with kidney function that their bodies are no longer able to excrete wastes in sufficient quantity to sustain a healthy body. This condition can be caused by a variety of diseases and can be so severe that a kidney transplant is required, or can be transient, related to another disease condition, such as a crisis in sickle cell anemia.

When the kidneys, for whatever reason, fail to function, death will occur in a brief period of time if no therapy is instituted. One palliative therapy that has literally been a life saver for many whose kidneys have failed is dialysis. What the dialysis machine does, in essence, is to take over the tasks of the kidneys, particularly in filtering and cleansing the blood. Dialysis may be either short- or long-term, depending upon the underlying cause of the kidney failure, and can keep a patient alive until a kidney transplant can be done, if that is possible or appropriate. Dialysis is an expensive, time consuming process, and must be repeated at least weekly and sometimes as often as daily or every other day. Some hospitals provide this service on either an ambulatory or inpatient basis. There are also independent, freestanding dialysis centers in some communities, and some patients have home dialysis setups for long-term care.

Surgery has been discussed as a curative therapy, but it can also be used as a palliative measure. The patient who is suffering from terminal cancer and experiences bowel obstruction from metastasis (spreading) of the cancer can have surgery to relieve the obstruction as a palliative treatment. A colostomy would probably be performed to bypass the obstruction and provide relief for the patient and possibly extend life for a period of time, also preventing what might well be a horrible, painful, and slow death from the obstruction. Another example of palliative surgery is the deadening or severing of nerve endings that cause chronic pain to a paralyzed patient or one with terminal cancer. Surgery for relief of pain for any reason can be termed a palliative measure because it does not *cure* the underlying cause of the pain, but provides *relief* from chronic pain. Many of the therapies already discussed and those to follow overlap in function and purpose.

Medications can be both curative and palliative. The use of medication as palliative therapy is different from the chemotherapy already discussed. Whereas the drugs used in chemotherapy are antineoplastic preparations, the drugs we are referring to here are in the families of the analgesics or pain relief categories. Narcotics are used singly or in combination with tranquilizers and/or other drugs to provide pain relief and comfort to patients, and are palliative rather than curative measures. Drugs used as comfort measures for patients are quite varied and almost all patients receive some form of pain medication during a typical hospital stay.

Other patients, with terminal illnesses, can receive doses of pain killing drugs far beyond what might be termed therapeutic. There are devices that can be used in these instances to automatically inject doses of palliative pain killers at regular intervals.

Custodial Therapy

Intravenous therapy, or IV therapy, is a form of custodial therapy that many hospital patients have experienced at one time or another. Any patient who requires fluid and electrolyte management will receive intravenous therapy. This includes virtually all patients undergoing surgery.

There are many instances when patients must be kept NPO, that is, having "nothing by mouth" for a period of time. Postoperatively, a patient may be kept NPO for 1 or more days in order to allow gastrointestinal function to return to normal. With intravenous therapy, there is no cause for alarm, as all basic fluid and electrolyte needs can be met for a short period of time with no harm to the patient. Of course, over the long term, intravenous therapy cannot fulfill all the required nutritional needs.

Intravenous solutions are incredibly varied and too numerous to list, but one solution widely used is dextrose in water. Sometimes medications (such as antibiotics) are added to the solution. In this case, the intravenous then may move into the cure arena if, in fact, the disease the patient is suffering from is an infection and the cure is antibiotic therapy. Vitamins may also be added to supplement the patient's needs. These are only two examples, however, of the many medications that might be added to intravenous solutions or given in what is called an intravenous push in a concentrated amount.

Many hospitals employ intravenous therapists to oversee all use of intravenous solution and take responsibility for starting all intravenous lines. Other hospitals do not have this service and rely on the physicians and nurses to provide this therapy. Physicians may start the intravenous lines, but the nurses are virtually always the ones to monitor the solutions, change bottles or bags of solution, and so on. In some hospitals, all medications added to intravenous solution are added and mixed by the pharmacists.

Blood transfusions are a form of widely used therapy for those who have suffered blood loss in trauma, surgery, or through illness. Blood transfusion therapy has made possible the recent advances in surgery we have all come to rely upon. Without the availability of blood, and the typing and cross-matching to minimize the problem of untoward reaction to the blood, surgery, especially that with a risk for significant blood loss, would not be possible.

Blood transfusion therapy comes in a variety of forms. One can receive whole blood, packed cells, platelets, plasma, and other separate blood components. There are even artificial blood substitutes for those whose religious beliefs preclude transfusion of human blood.

Some persons require periodic blood transfusions to sustain life. Examples would be patients with Cooley's anemia or thalassemia and those with hemophilia.

Total parenteral nutrition (TPN) is used when patients require a nutritionally complete therapy delivered intravenously. Usually the jugular or subclavian vein is used. For the past several years, this form of nutrition therapy has been used for patients suffering from a wide variety of conditions that necessitate routes other than a tube directly into the stomach for tube feeding (gastrostomy), a nasogastric tube for the same purpose, or short-term intravenous fluid and electrolyte therapy.

Before the advent of this therapy, many patients died because of nutritional imbalance and deficiency. Patients who require this kind of custodial care include those with extensive inflammatory bowel conditions; burn victims; persons undergoing chemotherapy; and malnourished persons with assorted problems, including anorexia, who cannot or will not eat.

In this chapter, we have attempted to describe several of the services offered in hospitals under the categories of diagnosis, cure, palliative measures, and custodial therapy. In the next chapter, we will focus on settings for hospital services, both outpatient and inpatient.

4

Settings for Hospital Services

Although we tend to think of hospitals as offering only inpatient residential care, it should now be evident that they provide services not only to those persons who are hospitalized or actually stay within the confines of the hospital walls 24 hours or longer, but to many persons who return to their own places of residence once they have received care, and return to the hospital as necessary on an ambulatory or day care basis. In this chapter, we will discuss both outpatient and inpatient services that a hospital might offer.

OUTPATIENT SERVICES

Ambulatory Care

Ambulatory Surgery. One of the services that hospitals are beginning to offer more frequently under the umbrella of ambulatory services is ambulatory surgery, more commonly referred to as same day or day surgery. For this care, the patient is never hospitalized overnight. All the preoperative preparations such as blood work, urinalysis, x-rays, and electrocardiogram are done on an outpatient basis a day or more before the scheduled surgery or on the day of surgery.

The person arrives at the hospital at the designated time on the day of surgery, not having eaten or taken anything by mouth since midnight of the previous day, and is prepared for surgery upon arrival. The patient changes into a surgical gown referred to as a "johnny." This garment generally ties in the back and is approximately knee length. A wrist identification band with all the necessary information is applied, much the same as with admission to the hospital. Preoperative medications may be given and the patient is taken by wheelchair or stretcher to surgery. If the surgery is scheduled later in the day, preoperative medication may be delayed until an appropriate time, and the patient waits in a preoperative area either in bed or in a lounge chair. In this case, the patient is usually given a robe and slippers to wear.

All the same procedures are followed as with any other surgical patient. The only exception is the fact that, once recovered from anesthesia either in the recovery room or more usually in a day surgery ward, the patient will return home that same day.

The trend toward day surgery has met with considerable success. Financially, 1-day surgery helps control the enormous cost of surgical care. The development of new techniques and recent advancements in medicine and surgery have made it a safe alternative. Some surgery performed on a day surgery basis includes biopsies; cosmetic procedures; dental extractions; arthroscopic exams; and many gynecologic techniques, such as dilatation and curretage (D & C) of the uterus, and laparoscopy.

In addition to the financial savings, there is also a psychological benefit to the patients using this service. Parents of small children with no responsible adult to care for their children during hospitalization are greatly relieved by this service. For others, for whom the time away from job or home would cause them to delay seeking treatment because of overnight hospitalization, an alternative is now available. Children can now return to the more familiar home environment without having the trauma of hospitalization added to the trauma of surgery. Ambulatory surgery also seems, for some persons, to lessen the emotional stress that is added to the usual anxieties of impending anesthesia and surgery. For those who take advantage of day surgery, the experience is very positive generally and viewed as extremely beneficial for all concerned.

Outpatient Clinics. Outpatient services are another kind of service provided under ambulatory care. As we discussed in an earlier chapter, the hospital outpatient department can serve as the primary care provider or primary health care provider for individuals. Depending upon the particular hospital, staff, and orientation of the hospital, outpatient clinics may be available for a wide variety of general and specialized services. Some of these require appointments and others will literally provide walk-in service. It is safe to say that there is an outpatient clinic for almost every specialty or subspecialty in one hospital or other and, in a large city, virtually all services are available somewhere on an outpatient basis. For example, one hospital may offer a clinic service that deals with correction of facial deformities, whereas another will offer a sleep disorder or headache clinic. The research being done at a particular hospital often determines which clinics are available, as will the residency training programs in specialty areas such as gynecology, obstetrics, orthopedics, pediatrics, neurology, and so on.

Clinics serving a larger segment of the population than specialties are available in many if not most hospitals, except those community hospitals affiliated only with physicians in private practice. Examples of common clinics include general medical and surgical clinics, pediatrics, gynecology, and orthopedics. Sports medicine has become a recent addition to many hospital outpatient services because of the interest seen today in exercise and physical fitness.

Alcohol and substance abuse clinics are also on the increase, as is the availability of psychiatric mental health services. Other examples of outpatient services include blood pressure, diabetes, prenatal, and family planning clinics. While clinics such as cystic fibrosis, parasitology, muscular dystrophy, and multiple sclerosis serve a more select population and may be found only in specialty hospitals or teaching hospitals, they may serve as referral centers for other institutions. Enterostomal and eating disorder clinics are also increasing in number, and appear in more community hospitals as well as in large urban medical centers. Esoteric services, such as in vitro fertilization programs, continue to be the exception and are found only in regional or teaching hospital settings.

Some large urban hospitals have added travel clinics to accommodate those who are bound for distant lands. A complete program from inoculations, treatment, and prescriptions for endemic conditions, as well as information and advice on how to avoid illness and disease, is available.

Women's health service is another example of a need expressed by a community that is now being met by some hospital outpatient services. The whole gamut of care for women, from routine Pap smears and pelvic examinations to gynecologic counseling, birth control, infertility work-ups, childbirth care, and sexual assault counseling and intervention, can be available. The staff can include nurse midwives, nurse practitioners, and physicians.

Support Group Services. Support group services are another form of ambulatory care that hospitals have recognized as needed and are now offering to their communities. Many of these are part of the social services department and meet at the hospital once or twice a month or more, if needed.

There are support groups for almost any area where it is therapeutic for those involved, whether for the patient, the family, and/or significant others, to come together as a group to share difficulties and support each other through trying times. The leader or support person is often a social worker or other health care professional who acts as facilitator and guides the group.

The idea of a support group can be thought of as vital to the adjustment and acceptance of those faced with problems or illnesses, or for their loved ones. Some of the support groups available include: Alzheimer's disease, arthritis, child abuse, sudden infant death syndrome (SIDS, crib death), cancer, ostomy, and diabetes. Some hospitals have begun to include spouse bereavement groups and overeaters anonymous as well. Whenever a need arises, a group can be formed to provide the necessary support, and usually the hospital staff is most receptive to any and all ideas.

Ambulatory Oncology Services. Ambulatory oncology services are offered by outpatient departments to the community and sometimes even to a region. The patient needing oncology treatment, therefore, does not need to be an inpatient to receive the chemotherapy, radiation, or whatever treatment is ongoing. In fact, this is often a much more positive approach to service for an oncology patient. The patient does not have to alter her/his lifestyle any more than for the time necessary to complete an individual treatment.

The oncology service is usually comprised of physicians, nurses, nurse practitioners, social workers, dieticians, and other health care professionals who make up a truly interdisciplinary team. The focus of care is to select and provide the treatment necessary to combat the malignancy and prevent metastasis or recurrence. There may be a combination of treatments or just one form.

The patient and family/significant others are brought into the discussion and a decision is reached jointly as to the best possible treatment for the disease and the optimal schedule for completion of the treatment. The staff takes a very personal approach when providing cancer therapy and develops considerable rapport with these patients. The emotional component can be very therapeutic to patients receiving cancer therapy, and the fact that they can remain at home while receiving treatment is an added bonus.

Miscellaneous Services. Under the heading of services provided on an outpatient basis that can be part of the offerings of a hospital to the community at large are a host of other programs that, for lack of a better category, can be termed miscellaneous. These include periodic screening clinics such as glaucoma, blood pressure, and diabetes; education classes for childbirth, parenting, diabetes self care, and exercise and weight maintenance; rape crisis, sexual assault, child sexual abuse, and domestic violence programs including hot lines; smoking cessation clinics; baby sitter training programs; physician referral registries; speakers bureau; community agency referral services; and outreach programs for the community at large, such as an immunization van or health fair. Some hospitals have a telephone number one can call to request information about dozens of conditions. A tape describing the condition, what to do, programs available, and so on is then played. Topics range from prevention of heart attack to the development of a 2-year-old. Some hospitals have a library and/or gift shop run by volunteers that can serve the inpatients, staff, visitors, and even the community at large. Some have a cafeteria or snack bar for visitors, staff, and outpatients and even provide nutrition education as part of the service. Hospital chapels are not uncommon, especially in hospitals sponsored by a religious group, and these are often open to persons in the community as well as to those in the hospital. CPR (cardiopulmonary resuscitation) training and first aid classes are offered by some institutions. Teenagers in the community can volunteer to be "candy stripers" (the name comes from their red-and-white striped uniforms) and learn firsthand what goes on in the hospital. A barber shop and/or hairdresser can also be available for patients and even occasionally for staff needs on a fee-for-service basis. In some ways, a hospital is like a small community, with all sorts of services available to its residents, sometimes its employees, and even the community at large.

Day Care. This is a service that some hospitals are now providing for two segments of the population. Some hospitals now sponsor day care centers within the hospital grounds for children of employees. The day care center can also be open to the community at large for child care for a fee. Places of employment that provide on-site day care find that employees are absent less frequently and are more conscientious workers when their children are nearby and their child care needs settled.

A second kind of day care that some hospitals are now providing to their communities is elder day care. With the ever growing population of older adults in the community who are able to live independently and yet require some services and support to keep them in their homes or in the homes of family members, these elder day care programs are essential. The broad range of services offered includes some nursing care; social services of all types; physical, occupational, and speech therapy; and nutrition. The older adult client needs to be with others and to be stimulated mentally and physically. Isolation can bring about deterioration and despair.

In day care, the elderly person enjoys the company of others while a staff of health care professionals administers to his/her individual needs. The day care members usually arrive in the morning with a family member or by elder transportation services and return home by dinner time. All meals are provided during the daytime hours and are eaten in a restaurant-like group setting. The atmosphere is one of congeniality and the food is prepared not only to appeal, but to meet the nutritional requirements of each individual.

For many older adults, day care gives them the best of both worlds. They are actively cared for during the day by a host of gerontology expert providers and are still able to live at home alone or with family members. Family members are relieved of the responsibility of care during the day when they are at work or busy with other responsibilities, such as small children, or are unable to provide all the care because of their own physical limitations.

Maintaining an optimal level of health and well-being is the goal of elder day care. Prior to the advent of this day care, many older adults were placed in nursing homes and other similar facilities or deteriorated at home alone with no one to care. This service has given them the freedom to remain at home for as long as possible and be truly well cared for. Keeping the mind and body active enables these folks to be free from being alone all day and gives them a purposeful sense of living.

At day care, group discussions are encouraged, events such as birthdays are celebrated, and many other therapeutic and recreational activities are provided. The discussion of current events helps keep everyone alert and participating, and other newsworthy conversation is shared and encouraged by all.

The programs are flexible. Those who can walk are encouraged to do so out of doors whenever possible, and a varied routine, from exercise to tips on how to keep healthy, is provided. There is, of course, access to medical care and assorted therapies when needed.

These elder day care centers benefit not only the older adult client who lives alone, but also those who live with relatives who are away at work all day. Knowing that their loved ones are being stimulated and cared for while they are away reduces the guilt many families have about the elderly member who would otherwise be home alone counting the hours until they return. The centers also make available health care professionals who can continually assess the individual's capacity and help maintain abilities for as long as possible.

INPATIENT SERVICES

Residential Inpatient Care

This section will be devoted to a discussion of the hospital setting and the typical hospital routine that is experienced by the patient and by the professional health care providers who practice in and are employed by hospitals. Most large urban hospitals resemble any high rise apartment complex and differ sharply in appearance from their suburban and community hospital counterparts. What goes on inside, however, and the general formula or layout, can be quite similar.

As one enters the building, there is usually an information desk or communication center where all visitor and patient information is dispensed. Flowers are often delivered to this desk and even mail as well, although in a very large medical center there will probably be a mail room and even a mail delivery truck dock. Sometimes, adjacent to the information desk or counter, there is a communication room with a switchboard and paging system, and today it is common to see one or more computer terminals.

The admitting office is usually off to one side, although in very large hospitals it may be on another floor. The admitting area resembles any private office space, where a typist sits on one side of the desk gathering information and the patient is on the other. Usually pertinent information regarding medical insurance, next of kin, employment, and other vital statistics is asked of the patient, and then an identifying bracelet is put on the person. The bracelet typically contains the following information: the patient's name, physician, hospital assigned number, and date of admission.

The patient is often asked to read and sign a general consent form. This is a consent for admission to and treatment in that hospital and may include a surgical consent form as well, if surgery is planned. More often today, the surgical consent and anesthesia permission forms are signed the evening before the scheduled surgery.

Once the paperwork is completed, the patient is taken to the assigned hospital room for further admission work. Sometimes volunteers from the hospital auxiliary escort patients to their rooms and at other times, a transport aide takes over.

The patient care units are very similar from one hospital to another. The layout may differ slightly, depending upon the interior design of the hospital and its age. The standard format is for patient rooms, containing one, two, three, or four beds, to run along a corridor and be numbered. The nurses' station may precede the rooms along the hall or, if there are two parallel halls, a short connecting corridor may contain the nurses' station. In a variation on this, the nurses' station is at the apex of a "v" and two corridors of patient rooms form the sides of the "v." In a round building, the nurses' station is in the center and the patient rooms run around the periphery.

The nurses' station is the central office area where the patients' charts, the kardex (a card file of patients), and other items pertaining to the organization of patient care are kept. For example, the physicians' order book and all nursing care assignments would be found in the nurses' station. Other items might include: nurses' time sheets (when they are scheduled to work); laboratory and x-ray request forms;

patient charge slips for items that must be individually charged and a machine to do the charges similar to a credit card machine at a store; all office supplies and paper; all forms that pertain to the work of all employees on the unit; all supplies used to record patient progress and care; procedure books; the hospital pharmacy directory; diet manual; pertinent textbooks; a drug directory or handbook (often the PDR: the physician's desk reference, an annual listing of available pharmaceutical products); and many other items too numerous to list. Those items needed for patient care that are not found in the nurses' station are either in the utility room, a storage room, or closet; the medicine closet, room, or cart; linen closet or cart; and unit kitchen, if one exists. All special pieces of equipment and supplies used only occasionally come from other parts of the hospital, including housekeeping, central supply, the pharmacy, maintenance, and direct from purchasing.

It is in the nurses' station where all patient calls from their call buttons, call lights, or intercoms are heard or seen and registered. Sometimes the room number lights up on a board, a flashing lighted number appears on a screen, a buzzing sound occurs, or the patient can actually speak through the intercom to state the need. There are different sounds made by emergency calls, and the ear becomes trained to them very quickly once they are part of one's everyday world.

In the kardex is the vital information about each patient, such as: medical and nursing diagnoses, next of kin, age, physician, religion, diet, home address, and nursing care plan. This nursing care plan is prepared by the primary nurse or the admitting nurse, and outlines the care required by the patient. The written plan assures follow-up (when the primary nurse is not at work) and continuity from one shift to another. All medications are listed and the times they are to be administered. All treatments and how they are to be performed should be clearly stated, as should the times at which they are to be done. A nurse new to the unit should be able to look at the kardex and get a brief profile of each patient and a total picture of the care he/she requires over a 24-hour period. If the patient has a special condition affecting care, *that* should also be noted, such as being hard of hearing or blind, so that those providing care will be aware of special needs. The kardex to be useful must be up-to-date, of course, and a new nursing care plan is prepared each time a major event, such as surgery, occurs.

The physicians' order book contains all the orders written for a particular patient by the attending and any consulting physicians. Sometimes the order sheets are kept in the patients' charts rather than in a single book. Medication orders are generally written on a separate form with several carbons, one of which goes to the pharmacy. The pharmacist fills the orders directly, rather than from someone else's copy (and possibly erroneous interpretation) of what was originally written. Those caring for patients refer to the physicians' order sheets and medication orders for any changes in or questions about medical care. Some of the care given by nurses is medical care that the nurse administers, such as giving the patient medications the physician has ordered. Other care is nursing care individually designed to promote comfort, prevent complications, promote healing, teach the patient and/or family about any care they will be giving after discharge, and return the patient to the highest possible level of wellness.

Many of the questions a care giver might have about a particular patient can be answered in the nurses' station. For example, if a nurse is unsure of the medication that is ordered, she/he can look it up in a pharmacy reference work, the hospital formulary, or call up the pharmacy.

Many hospitals have procedure manuals, explaining the hospital's protocol for certain treatments, the equipment available, and the steps to be followed. Since hospitals vary on some procedures, such as the type of enema equipment available, the procedure book can be very useful. What is most important is that the procedure be done correctly so that the desired effect is accomplished; that the patient's safety, privacy, and comfort be protected; and that protection from trauma or infection be assured. Procedures are intended to do these things. Some hospitals use a standardized procedure text and make their own modifications.

The diet manual is a great aid in checking which foods are prohibited from certain types of diets and which ones are allowed. No one can be expected to remember every detail about every diet, and the manual serves as a wonderful reference. Some hospitals produce their own manuals and others use a published reference work.

In addition to the nurses' station, all nursing units have a clean utility room, a dirty utility room, linen closets or carts or rooms, and a general storage area of some sort for equipment used all the time, like portable intravenous (IV) poles, scales, wheelchairs, stretchers, suction machines, and so on. The nature of the equipment will, of course, be determined by the type of patients cared for on the unit. Every unit has some sort of utility area for the housekeeping personnel as well, where mops, pails, soap, disinfectant solutions, and so on are kept.

The clean utility room contains all the sterilized and packaged supplies and equipment needed on a medical, surgical, or specialty unit. All prepacked, clean and sterile equipment is also found here, as well as items such as wash basins, bedpans, soap, and backrub lotion. Virtually any items needed for patient care, except linen and medications, would be kept in the clean utility room.

In the dirty utility room are the refuse cans for disposing of used equipment such as empty intravenous bottles or bags and tubing, and sink areas for rinsing equipment that has been used. A bedpan sterilizer is also located in the dirty utility room. This unit, referred to as a "hopper," flushes and sterilizes any bedpan. This is a particularly useful item when the patient rooms do not have individual bathrooms. Urine testing and collection of urine and stool specimens is also done in the dirty utility room.

Some nursing units have small kitchens or kitchen areas. These generally contain an ice machine and a refrigerator for beverages for patients and snacks for the afternoon and evening. Depending upon the procedure for delivery of meal trays to patients, the kitchen may also serve as a holding area for trays, with a dumbwaiter that conveys trays to and from the central kitchen. There may be a stove or burner unit complete with kettle for making tea or other hot beverages, should a patient request one. Occasionally, there is a toaster and even a microwave oven, but this is not the usual equipment found in all kitchen areas.

Most meal trays come to nursing units in a hot food serving cart and are passed to each patient by either the unit staff members or a dietary aide. Sometimes volunteers, like teenage candy stripers, help to serve the trays. When a patient is in isolation, the nursing staff is generally responsible for delivery and retrieval of meals and equipment, since special procedures must be followed.

The linen closets, rooms, or carts are used to store linen not used for morning care, but available for use should the need arise. Linen carts are often delivered to each floor each day or twice a day, and what remains unused is stored in the closets for the other shifts to use and the cart is returned to the central linen room.

The linen for a typical patient unit consists of bed sheets, one of which may be contour; drawsheets, which are half sheets used cross-wise over the bottom sheet to provide extra absorbency; and a pillow case. Sometimes a disposable wet-proof pad is placed under the drawsheet and then only this pad and the drawsheet need to be changed throughout the day if they become soiled or wet. Drawsheets are also helpful for moving and lifting patients. Untucking the sides and rolling the ends toward the middle and pulling toward the head of the bed, with another person doing the same on the other side, is a great aid in helping immobile patients get into a better position. The drawsheet can also be used to turn the patient or to position her/him on either side.

In addition to sheets of all sorts, there are bath blankets, made of a soft flannelette used to ward off the chill when bathing a patient. The bath blanket also protects the patient from being exposed during the bath and absorbs any excess moisture that would otherwise wet the bed. Some hospitals also have cotton thermal bed blankets and bedspreads available.

Face and bath towels, washcloths, and "johnny gowns" (described earlier) are supplied for each patient. Other items are robes, pajama bottoms with drawstring waists, and sheepskin pads for the bed to prevent bedsores. Sometimes the linen is in pastel colors rather than white to detract from the sterile atmosphere and more closely resemble home.

In keeping with this idea, the trend is to have patient rooms painted or papered in soft colors or restful patterns and sometimes to include artwork or other wall decorations to simulate a more home-like atmosphere. Curtains and furnishings such as chairs tend to be more home-like as well, compared with past years.

The basic patient room consists of the assigned number of beds and often an adjoining bathroom containing a sink and toilet. Within the room is the requisite number of closets; bureaus or built-in bureau drawers; and bedside and overbed tables for each bed. Generally, only the television set and the bathroom are shared in a multipatient room, although now with mini television sets, each patient may have one.

Above each bed is a light fixture and wall equipment for oxygen, suction, and blood pressure, although older hospitals may not have this equipment built in as yet. There is a call light connected by a cord and attached to the bed so the patient can be in contact with the nurses' station. There is also an emergency call button in the bathroom for the same purpose. Some hospitals also have intercom systems.

At the bedside, there is a nightstand that contains a wash basin, soap dish, emesis basin, urinal (for males), and a bedpan. Today, these are often disposable items and the patient can take them home on discharge. In the nightstand, there is a drawer for personal items and toiletries. Sometimes there is a thermometer and holder, depending upon the equipment used in a particular hospital. Many now use digital thermometer equipment on all patients. A water pitcher and glass are left on top of the nightstand so the patient can drink at will, except when NPO.

The overbed table can be raised or lowered as desired and serves as a tray table for meals, whether the patient is in bed or seated in a chair. It is also used as a stand for the wash basin when the patient bathes in bed. Some overbed tables have an adjustable mirror that can be pulled from the top and angled to benefit the bedbound patient in shaving and grooming. This mirror folds flat when not in use so the table can be used for other purposes.

The hospital generally provides soap, tissues, and toilet paper, but rarely a toothbrush and toothpaste. The patient must bring deodorant and comb from home, although the gift shop often sells these items for those who forget them. Food and linens are included in the room rate, but any other items used in care, such as an enema set, are charged separately to the patient, as are all medications.

Patient rooms generally have one or more comfortable chairs for patient and visitor use, and often a straight chair or two as well. Beds today are usually electric-powered, allowing the bed to be kept at normal bed height for ease in getting in and out, and elevated when the patient is receiving care such as a bed bath. The controls are within easy reach of the patient and make it possible for her/him to raise and lower the head and foot at will. If there is more than one bed in the room, the beds are separated by curtains that surround each bed to provide privacy and can be pulled to one side when not in use.

The telephone is generally, although not always, shared, or the hospital may have a policy of putting in a telephone only at the request of the patient. Showers are available either in individual patient bathrooms or in a shower room down the corridor, but generally patients must have permission for all sorts of activity, including showering and walking around the unit. Bathtubs are generally not found in hospitals, for safety reasons and because they would be very difficult to clean between patients.

Floors in patient areas today are sometimes carpeted or the patient rooms may have tile floors and the corridors and nurses' station have carpeting. The floors are kept meticulously clean and, if tile, are generally washed and polished daily. Sometimes there is a patient or visitor lounge on the unit with comfortable chairs, perhaps a television, and sometimes carpeting. Some units even have a lounge area with tables where ambulatory patients can have their meals. There may be a conference room where nurses and other health care professionals can hold meetings out of the mainstream of patient and traffic flow. This room can also be used for teaching patients, either individually or in groups, and may be equipped with a blackboard, screen, and other teaching materials.

The Hospital Routine

Hospital routine will vary slightly, depending upon the hospital and the type of unit, but generally it is pretty much the same. The nursing staff is assigned to rotating shifts. The shifts are from 7:00 a.m. to 3:00 or 3:30 p.m., 3:00 p.m. to 11:00 or 11:30 p.m., and 11:00 p.m. to 7:00 a.m. There are variations, but shifts are generally 8 or 8½ hours in length. Some hospitals are trying 10-hour shifts for certain patient areas, so that the nursing staff works 4 days a week instead of 5. Many of the staff rotate between two shifts and others may have a permanent shift to work. Generally, nursing staff members know at least 2 weeks in advance of their scheduled shifts and hours at work, as well as their days off for that period of time. Working weekends is the norm, with some hospitals attempting to give staff every other or every third weekend off. Some hospitals have part-timers who work only weekends and these persons are very helpful in offering full-time staff members time off. The head nurse of a unit generally works every other weekend. Because nurses are responsible for care 24 hours a day, 7 days a week, working around the clock and on weekends and holidays is part of the commitment of the profession.

Each day shift begins with receiving report from the night staff. Often the report is taped, so that the night nurses can complete their responsibilities and go home on time and the day staff can refer to the taped report as often as they wish. What the report entails is a brief summary of how each patient spent the night. Details of impending surgery, tests, admissions, and discharges and so on are discussed, so that everyone is informed. The day staff thus can plan their care to meet the patients' needs and accommodate care giving to tests, trips to x-ray, physical therapy, surgery, and whatever else is planned.

If the report is not taped, it is the responsibility of the nurse in charge of the night shift to give the report orally when incoming staff has congregated together. Then the day staff will meet briefly to discuss assignments and care plans.

Breakfast is served around 8:00 a.m. and vital signs are taken just prior to the passing of the diet trays. While the patients are eating, the staff plans their day, gathers the necessary linen, and prepares for giving morning care to their patients. Morning medications may be given by the nurse caring for the patient or by a medication nurse, depending upon hospital policy. Each individual nurse is responsible for the medications all of her/his patients are receiving if primary nursing is a model for practice.

Morning care consists of a complete bath given by the nurse or a partial bath in which the nurse assists the patient in bathing. Sometimes a patient will take a shower or sponge bath alone in the bathroom and wish to assume total care. Patients who are confined to bedrest generally appreciate a bed bath and the nurse can assess the skin and perform a range of motion exercises that are beneficial to the patient, as well as giving a backrub.

The patient's private physician will visit sometime during the day, often during the morning hours, and if the hospital is a teaching institution, morning or afternoon rounds are held. This means that, in addition to the private physician, if the patient has one, the interns, residents, and medical students will examine the patient and discuss his/her condition and treatment. Physician visits and teaching rounds often occur without any notice, so nursing staff learn to accommodate the care they are giving patients to this interruption. In many hospitals, nurses make separate nursing rounds and/or are part of teaching rounds with the physicians.

All ordered medical and nursing treatments and health teaching are included in the morning care, as well as at other times of the day, when appropriate. The nurse and patient interact throughout the morning and work at establishing rapport with each other. If primary nursing is practiced, the patient has one nurse to relate to for all the important care and teaching.

Should the patient be scheduled for x-rays, physical therapy, or other diagnostic or therapeutic interventions that take

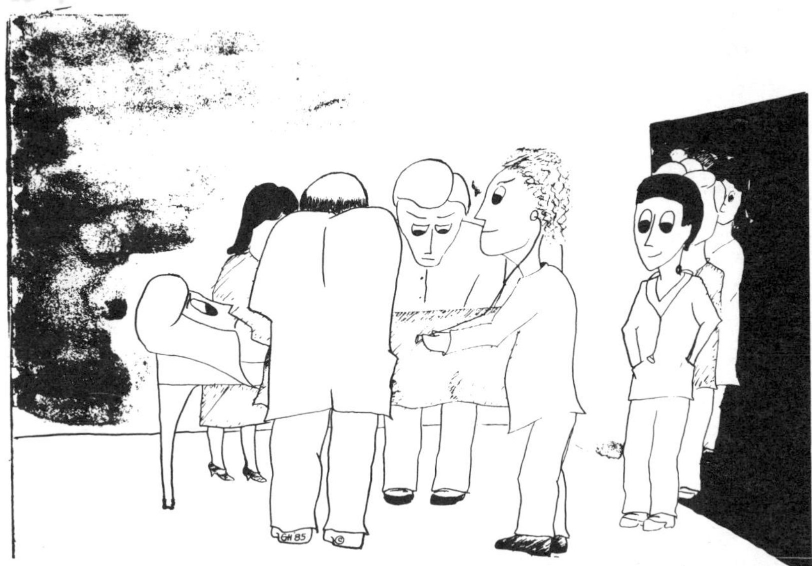

Figure 4.1 Why is it patients seem to need to be seen by two dozen persons a day? (© Glen D. Hawkins).

place off the unit, the particular department will call for the patient at the prescribed time and return him/her to the room. Some hospitals have transport aides who do all the transporting of patients to and from every area of the hospital, and then arrangements are made for the transport through a central service. Sometimes it is also the responsibility of the nurse caring for the patient to do the transporting.

In addition to visits by medical staff, pastoral staff may visit as well. Patients find comfort in having members of the pastoral counseling service visit and often seem to welcome these persons. Of course, a patient also has the right to refuse any visitors. The patient's own clergy are also welcome to visit and hospitals of any denomination are open to ministers, priests, rabbis, and clergy of any religious orientation to visit their parish members.

Before too long, the morning is past and it is time for noon vital signs on those patients needing more than once-a-day monitoring; urine testing for patients with diabetes; medications; and lunch. Visiting hours vary, but generally are from 1:00 p.m. to 8:00 p.m. For certain units, visiting hours are more restricted, and for others, more liberal, such as 24 hours a day for fathers in the maternity unit. Most patients welcome visitors, especially family, and look forward to visiting hours. Some even look perkier and are more animated when surrounded by loved ones. It is obviously important for nurses to pay attention to the effects visitors have on patients and to intervene, when appropriate, to protect the patient's well-being or to suggest that family visit more often if someone is always alone.

Some patients catnap in the afternoon, while others read or watch television or simply ambulate in the hallways or lounge. For the very ill patients, confined to bedrest, time of day does not seem very important, and their care and monitoring continues throughout the day.

Nurses usually have a short break in the morning and a lunch time lasting about 30 minutes. Lunch is usually eaten in the hospital cafeteria, but many hospitals have a coffee shop that provides an alternative. Many nurses brown bag it, while others have their main meal of the day at lunchtime. Students usually have cafeteria privileges and some also choose to bring a lunch and eat in the nurses' lounge area. All foods are prepared and served attractively in hospital cafeterias and provide wholesome nutrition. Salad bars have become quite a popular addition to hospital cafeterias, and many of the staff opt for a green salad for lunch. Fresh fruit and yogurt are generally available as an alternative to hot meals and sandwiches. Some hospital cafeterias are now offering nutrition information and education to staff and visitors, through labeling of foods offered as to nutritional value, pamphlets, signs, and sample menus. Very often the cafeteria is open for visitors to use as well, and many are grateful for the opportunity to stay within the hospital setting to eat. This is especially true for those who have spent long, stressful hours waiting for a family member to return from surgery.

After lunch, the nurses' hours are spent caring for patients, providing any necessary medications or treatments, and completing the charting of activities of the day, updating the care plan, and preparing the report for the next shift. Sometimes group classes are offered on topics such as pre- and postoperative care, diabetes self care, and nutrition. Closed circuit television is also used for patient instruction.

In a maternity unit, infant feedings are integrated around the infant's demands and a roughly every 4-hour schedule. Classes are frequently offered for the women on child care topics. Since the hospital stay is very brief, especially for women who have had a vaginal birth, much teaching is necessary to prepare the family to go home, both about care and feeding of the infant and the care the mother needs. The nursery is generally located on the same floor as the postpartum unit, so women can take their babies back and forth to the nursery if they are not having the infant room-in. The trend today is for nurses to be assigned to care for both mother and infant, unless the infant is in the special care nursery, which may even be located on another floor.

In a pediatric unit, there may be a playroom and a schoolroom where children who are able spend part of their day. Children who are hospitalized for long periods of time may also have tutors who come to their hospital rooms to help them keep up with their studies. Sometimes children are in play therapy in an area in another part of the hospital.

The change of shift for nurses comes around 3:00 p.m., unless the nurses are working 10-hour shifts, and the late afternoon routine begins: medications; treatments; communicating with patients; preoperative teaching; and preparations for surgery and for any tests scheduled for the next day. Visitors and supper complete the routine. Patients are often offered evening snacks or allowed to prepare their own in the unit kitchen. Supper can be served as early as 5:30 or 6:00 p.m., and it is a long time until breakfast!

The night shift is slightly different, in that many of the patients will sleep all night. Some women who are breast-feeding will feed their infants during the night, but many babies will be fed in the nursery. For those in need of constant care and vigilance, all hours are essentially the same and nursing care continues regardless of the time. Nursing satisfaction comes from being able to meet the needs of these patients and being there when visitors and other health care professionals are not. Generally at night, services such as laboratory, surgery, physical therapy, and so on are on an emergency basis only, so it is a time when nurses are the only ones giving care.

The routine of each hospital and each unit where you have your clinical experiences will vary from the description we have given you, of course. What we hope is that the information we have given you in this chapter will be useful in apprising you of what to expect and provoking you to seek information when you are uncertain. The next chapter is devoted to a description of the persons who are employed by and practice in a typical hospital.

5

Health Care Providers in the Hospital Setting

The number of health care providers in hospitals has mushroomed in the past several decades. From the dyad of nurse and physician of the 19th century have come specialties within these two professions and countless other professions, subspecialties, and paraprofessional groups. It has been said that "in health care, the individual has been replaced by a team of specialists who individually often do not know what the others are doing" (Bullough & Bullough, 1972, pp. 167–168). The health care industry as a whole is now the second largest employer of persons in this country. Of course, this means all the agencies, institutions, and businesses engaged in or having anything to do with health care, but nonetheless the figure is impressive. More than 30 occupations are now licensed in the health field in one or more states (Resources Administration, 1975, pp. 3–5). There are several million persons in health professions and occupations and more than two million allied health workers (aides, orderlies, ward clerks, technicians, and others). Many of these persons work in hospitals.

EDUCATION OF HEALTH CARE PROVIDERS

The educational level of health care workers reflects the same diversity as their titles. Levels of education range from less than elementary school to graduate degrees and post-graduate work. Nonprofessionals or allied health workers may receive on-the-job training or preparation in a trade school. Licensed practical or licensed vocational nurses are educated in hospital based, technical high school, or community college programs 1 to 2 years in length. Community colleges and technical schools also prepare laboratory assistants, respiratory therapists, dental technicians, and aides for physical therapy and other departments within the hospitals. These programs are 1 to 2 years in length and may be degree granting for 2 years (associate degree programs). Two-year associate degree programs also prepare individuals as nurses eligible to sit for the state licensing examinations and to use R.N. after their names, if they successfully complete the examinations.

Health care professionals are prepared at the baccalaureate, graduate degree, or professional school level. For example, nurses can complete a 4-year baccalaureate program in nursing or, if an individual holds a baccalaureate degree in another field, he or she can enroll in a master's program designed to prepare for beginning practice in nursing. Currently, there is also one nursing program which prepares the individual with the first nursing degree, a doctorate of nursing. Physical therapy; nutrition and dietetics; occupational therapy; laboratory technology; and some pharmacy programs grant a baccalaureate as the first professional degree. Pharmacy is moving rapidly to the equivalent of the master's degree, and social work education is now at the master's level and there are doctoral programs for advanced practice. There are graduate programs in nutrition, social work, speech therapy, physical and occupational therapy, and other health care professions, including nursing, as well, and the trend is toward more education for professional practice even at the entry level.

ROLES OF HEALTH CARE PROFESSIONALS IN THE HOSPITAL

Most health care providers are represented on the staffs of hospitals, although not in all hospitals. Smaller hospitals will, of course, have fewer employees and less specialization than will large institutions. Specialty hospitals employ specialists, just as their name implies. The sections to follow in this chapter will describe the major health care providers you will meet in a hospital and some of the specialists and subspecialists you may encounter during your years as a student and as a professional nurse or other health care professional.

Nurses

Nurses are the largest group of health care professionals in this country. There are approximately 1.4 million registered nurses holding active licenses to practice in the U.S.A. and 1.2 million are employed in nursing. The majority are women (95.6%), and the majority are married. About 6.2% are from minority groups. Most are employed in patient care settings and about 65% are working in hospitals (Statistical Abstract, 1984; ANA, 1981; NLN, 1982). Nurses provide most of the direct patient care in hospitals and are the health care professionals who spend the most time with patients. They are the 24-hour-a-day care providers 7 days a week. Nurses are generally employed by the hospital and may be either salaried employees or paid by the hour. Both part-time and full-time positions are generally available. Hospitals vary in their requirements for employment. Some will hire only graduates of baccalaureate or higher degree programs, whereas others will hire nurses from diploma and associate degree programs as well. Some hospitals will use licensed practical nurses and others will not. As nursing develops as a profession, more nurses with master's degrees and doctorates are available and hospitals are hiring these nurses for leadership positions, both in the provision of direct care to patients and also as administrators responsible for the care given by other nurses.

The structure of the nursing hierarchy also varies from hospital to hospital. Generally there is a director of nursing or a vice president for nursing as the chief administrative officer for nursing in the institution and then a number of

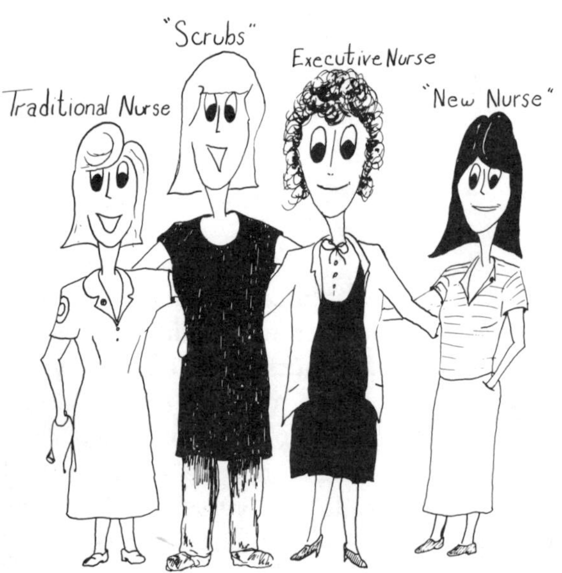

Figure 5.1 Types of nursing attire. (© Glen D. Hawkins).

associate directors. Some hospitals have supervisors responsible for one or more units or wards or specialty services, such as a supervisor for medical nursing, whereas others have clinical directors for services. Head nurses are used in some institutions to carry the administrative responsibilities for patient care on a floor, unit, or service, such as pediatrics, whereas other hospitals have clinical directors with these responsibilities.

Primary nursing is practiced in some settings. This form of organization for the delivery of nursing care allocates responsibility for the care of each patient in the hospital to one primary nurse and one or more associate nurses. The primary nurse has full 24-hour responsibility for giving and overseeing the nursing care given to her/his patients from admission to discharge. Other ways of organizing nursing care include team nursing, whereby a team of nurses assumes responsibility for a group of patients for a particular time period, and 1-to-1 assignment of patients to nurses, based on the patients and the nurses on duty during a particular time period. It is important to understand the organization of nursing care and administration in whatever hospital you are assigned as a student and are working in as a graduate.

Just as the organization of nursing varies from hospital to hospital, so do the responsibilities nurses carry for care of patients. In a large teaching hospital with many medical students, interns, and residents, nurses may have different responsibilities than in a small community hospital where there are only staff physicians. Also the number and variety of other health care professionals and providers available to give care to patients are greater, the larger and more diverse the hospital, so nurses will provide different kinds of care.

Nurses specialize in two different ways. The first is through on-the-job learning. The nurse who works for a time in an intensive care unit or in the newborn nursery or in pediatrics gains expertise from the experience in that unit. She/he should also be attending continuing education programs to increase her/his expertise in the area and be keeping current in the nursing literature. Specialization is also gained at the master's level of education when one selects a particular specialty for this advanced study (see table 5.1).

Whatever the structure and size of the hospital, however, nurses are responsible for most of the care patients receive during hospitalization. They are the day-to-day providers of care and must make decisions regarding the nursing care the patients are to receive and judgments as to when the expertise of other health care professionals is necessary. Part of your education will focus on assessing the condition of the patients for whom you care and making decisions concerning that care and the care to be given by others.

Physicians

Physicians in a hospital fall into two categories: 1) those employed by the hospital, and 2) those who are independent practitioners, but have privileges to practice in the hospital for those aspects of their practice requiring a hospital setting. We will first discuss the types of physicians who might be employed by a hospital and under which circumstances, and then we'll discuss the role of independent practitioners.

Certain types of hospitals employ virtually all the physicians practicing in those institutions. Military hospitals, those run by the federal government, and some state, county, and local hospitals may employ physicians on a salary basis much in the same way that they employ other health care professionals. These physicians work exclusively for that hospital or may share responsibilities with one or more other institutions, but are generally not in private practice on a fee-for-service basis elsewhere. Private hospitals sometimes employ physicians for certain special services, for example, anesthesiology; pathology; emergency room services; and ra-

TABLE 5.1 Specialization in Nursing

Administration	Specialist in nursing administration; administrative leadership of nursing in hospitals and community agencies
Adolescence	Care of adolescents in acute, ambulatory, or chronic care
Adult Nursing	Care of adults in acute, chronic, and/or ambulatory care settings
College Health	Care of students in the college and university setting
Community Health	Focus on the health of a community and its citizens
Family Health	Primary care of the family
Family Planning	Focus on care of women seeking fertility regulation
Gynecology	Care of women for those aspects unique to being a woman; concerns with the breasts and reproductive tract
Gerontology	Care of older adults
Maternal Child Health	Care of childbearing and childrearing families
Medical–Surgical	Care of adults with medical and surgical conditions; many nurses have subspecialties such as care of persons with cardiovascular; orthopedic; neurologic; eye; ear, nose, and throat; respiratory; renal; diabetic medical diagnoses; persons having organ transplants; persons in intensive care units
Neonatal	Care of newborn infants, especially those at high risk
Nurse Midwifery	Practice as a nurse midwife caring for pregnant, parturient, and postnatal women and their newborns (includes managing the labor and delivery)
Obstetrical	Care of pregnant, parturient, and postpartum women and their newborns; an alternate form of this is maternity
Occupational Health	Care of persons in the workplace
Parent/Child Nursing	Variation on the term maternal/child health; care of childbearing and childrearing families

TABLE 5.1 *(Continued)*

Pediatric	Care of children; subspecialties for children with renal, neurologic, cardiac, diabetic, or respiratory medical diagnoses; those having organ transplants; children with learning disorders, physical disabilities, and genetic anomalies
Perinatal	Care of pregnant women and their newborns
Psychiatric–Mental Health	Prevention of and care of persons with psychosocial concerns; subspecializations can be adults, adolescents, and children
School Health	Care of children and adolescents in school
Women's Health	Care of women across the life span; puberty to postmenopausal

diology. These physicians may or may not have a private practice in addition to their hospital responsibilities. This depends upon their arrangement with the hospital. Private hospitals may also be part of an intern and residency program under the aegis of a medical school and may, therefore, pay the salaries of those physicians in return for services to their patients. Medical centers with an affiliation with a medical school may also have arrangements for shared salaries with medical school faculty. The variety of possibilities for financial arrangements between hospitals and physicians is almost limitless.

Physicians in private, independent practice generally have what are known as staff privileges with one or more hospitals in order to be able to admit patients to the hospital and perform those procedures that necessitate hospital facilities. These physicians are not paid by the hospital, but rather collect their fees directly from patients for their services. In return for the use of the facilities of the hospital, the physician admits patients to the hospital and, therefore, provides the hospital with its income through charges to the patient for the room, as well as use of equipment, tests, therapeutic regimes, nursing care, and so on. Since physicians are often the only individuals authorized to admit patients to hospitals, hospitals depend upon them for their survival.

There are many specialties within medicine and subspecialties as well. Table 5.2 lists some of the major medical specialties. Many of these specialties will be represented on the staff of a moderate to large general hospital. A specialty hospital, such as a psychiatric or pediatric facility will, of course, have fewer specialties represented. And if there are a number of hospitals in a small geographic area, even general hospitals may choose not to offer every kind of service in order to save money on equipment and not duplicate services, so that providing care is cost-effective.

Other Health Care Professionals

There are many health care professionals in addition to nurses and physicians who may be employed in hospitals. The education and preparation of these persons vary with the field and with the individual requirements of the institution. Some of these individuals may be employed directly by the hospital and others may be employed elsewhere or in independent practice, the latter billing patients directly for their services. The larger the hospital, the more likely that the number and variety of health care professionals will be large.

Most hospitals of any size have a pharmacy staffed by one or more pharmacists. The physical and occupational therapy departments are staffed by professionals in those specialties. So are laboratories; speech and voice therapy; x-ray and other radiological services; the dietary service; social service; psychology; respiratory therapy; the medical records library; the medical and nursing reference libraries; anesthesia (which may have both physician anesthesiologists and nurse anesthetists); and the chaplaincy office. Some of these persons are, by definition, prepared at the master's level, and some

TABLE 5.2 Types of Physicians

Adolescent Medicine	Specialist in care and conditions of adolescents
Allergist	Diagnosis and treatment of conditions resulting from allergic responses
Anesthesiologist	Specialist in administration of all forms of anesthesia
Cardiologist	Diagnosis and treatment of conditions of the heart and blood vessels
Dermatologist	Diagnosis and treatment of diseases and conditions of the skin
Emergency Medicine	Diagnosis and treatment of emergency conditions such as trauma
Gastroenterologist	Diagnosis and treatment of conditions and diseases of the stomach, intestines, liver, pancreas, and gall bladder
Gerontologist	Specialist in the care and conditions of older adults
Gynecologist	Diagnosis and treatment of conditions and diseases of the woman's reproductive tract
Hematologist	Diagnosis and treatment of diseases and conditions of the blood and blood producing tissues of the body
Internal Medicine	Diagnosis and treatment of general medical conditions involving the internal organs; subspecialties might include diabetes, diseases of the digestive tract, rheumatology, gerontology, oncology, infectious diseases, allergy, endocrinology
Neurologist	Diagnosis and treatment of conditions and diseases of the nervous system
Neurosurgeon	Specialist in the surgical treatment of conditions of the brain, spinal cord, and nervous system
Nuclear Medicine	Specialist in the use of radioactive materials for diagnosis and treatment
Obstetrician	Diagnosis and care for women during and immediately following pregnancy
Ophthalmologist	Diagnosis and treatment of conditions and diseases of the eyes
Orthopedist	Specialization in the diagnosis and treatment of conditions and diseases of the bones, cartilage, ligaments, tendons, joints
Otolaryngologist	Diagnosis and treatment of conditions and diseases of the throat, nose, sinuses, and ears (referred to as ENT)
Pathologist	Study of tissues and cells
Pediatrician	Care of children

TABLE 5.2 *(Continued)*

Physical Medicine and Rehabilitation	Specialist in maintenance or restoration of abilities to perform activities of daily living following illness or injury, or related to a chronic condition
Preventive Medicine	Specialist in health prevention and maintenance strategies
Psychiatrist	Study and treatment of mental illness; subspecialties in adult and child psychiatry
Pulmonary	Diagnosis and treatment of conditions of the lungs
Radiologist	Specialist in x-ray and other radiological techniques for diagnosis and treatment
Sports Medicine	Specialist in conditions or injuries related to participation in sports
Surgeon	Specialist in performing surgical procedures; subspecialties in pediatric, urologic, gastrointestinal, neuro, gynecologic, plastic, thoracic, cardiac, pulmonary, ENT, orthopedic surgery
Urologist	Diagnosis and treatment of conditions and diseases of the urinary tract

at the baccalaureate or associate degree level. In fields such as social work, library science, physical and occupational therapy, and the clergy, some individuals will also hold an earned doctoral degree.

Of the 5,576,000 individuals employed in health occupations, pharmacists, dieticians, therapists (including occupational; physical; speech and hearing; and other professionals prepared at the baccalaureate or higher degree level), physicians' assistants, and managers comprise nearly 620,000. Health technicians and technologists, some of whom hold baccalaureate or higher degrees and some of whom have associate degrees or diplomas account for another 1,111,000 health care workers (Statistical Abstract, 1985, p. 102). Additionally, there are approximately 407,000 social workers in the United States, some of whom are directly employed by health care agencies and many of whom spend part of their time assisting clients with health-related needs (Statistical Abstract, 1985, p. 402).

Clinical dieticians hold a minimum of a baccalaureate degree. They are responsible for working with clients or selecting foods for them that will meet their particular nutritional needs. Dieticians use their knowledge of nutrition to teach clients, their families, and/or significant others, as well as other members of the health care team, about foods, food composition, and human needs (Mason, Wenberg, & Welsch, 1982). In some hospitals and other health care agencies, the clinical dietician oversees all aspects of the food service, including staff meals.

Physical therapists also hold a minimum of a baccalaureate degree. They are responsible for the diagnosis, plan, implementation, and evaluation of the patient's need for assistance with mobility. Their focus of concern can range from a single joint to the entire body, depending upon the extent of the body insult. This individual assists the patient to maintain or restore his or her capacity to undertake activities of daily living such as bathing, dressing, and household chores. The physical therapist utilizes specially adapted devices and equipment to augment the patient's abilities, such as specially constructed tableware, a raised toilet seat, and a seat in the shower. Physical therapists also assist other health care professionals to identify strategies that will enable the patient to achieve an optimal level of functioning of the musculoskeletal system. Their concerns include primary prevention, secondary intervention when a disease or injury has occurred, and tertiary prevention, the rehabilitative phase of care.

Closely allied to the work of the physical therapist is that of the *occupational therapist.* The occupational therapist assists the patient to reach and maintain an optimal level of functioning relative to that individual's role functioning. That is, the occupational therapist assists the homemaker to function with appropriate adaptations in his/her kitchen and household, the office person to be able to type, file, or whatever else is required in the position, and so on. Sometimes a home assessment is part of this person's role, in order to help the person to make appropriate adaptations to assure the highest degree of independence possible.

Pharmacists are prepared at the baccalaureate or higher degree level. They are responsible for all the drug needs of the patient in the hospital, and also work in ambulatory settings and other health care agencies. The pharmacist prepares prescriptions, dispenses medications to the patient units, stocks the units with those medications and solutions that are kept in bulk—such as antibacterials and over-the-counter analgesics and laxatives—and may also assume responsibility for adding medications to any intravenous solutions. He or she also may prepare all antineoplastic drugs and solutions.

Speech and hearing specialists are prepared at the baccalaureate or higher degree level. One individual may assist clients with both speech and hearing, or an individual may specialize in either speech or hearing disorders and their treatment. These professionals, as their titles imply, work with clients who have deficits in hearing or speaking, although the two may be interrelated, as in the case of a person who is deaf and, therefore, has difficulty learning to speak. The range of assessment, diagnosis, and intervention runs from the infant who has congenital deafness to the older adult whose speech is affected by a stroke.

Although *social workers* can receive their basic preparation at the baccalaureate level, the trend is for master's education for entry into the profession and for doctoral preparation for advanced practice and teaching. Social workers are concerned with many and diverse aspects of the social welfare of their clients. When employed by hospitals and other health care agencies and institutions, their responsibilities include assisting clients to understand and cope with the paperwork necessary to qualify for various third-party payers such as

Medicaid, Medicare, Veterans Administration, and other programs under the Social Security Administration; helping clients and their families and/or significant others to make decisions about health care; and identifying resources for basic needs such as food, heat, housing, clothing, and health care. Much time is spent in counseling clients who need assistance with decision making, coping with their own lives, and caring for children or older relatives.

Physicians' Assistants are relatively new members of the health care team. They work under the direction of physicians, performing some of the more repetitive tasks such as routine suturing of lacerations, setting uncomplicated fractures, and seeing clients for routine health maintenance and episodic acute care visits. Programs range in length from 1 to 2 years. Some programs require previous health care experience, such as being a registered nurse or having served in a military health corps. All require a preceptorship with a physician (Golden, 1979).

Members of the clergy may choose to serve as *hospital chaplains,* either through a chaplaincy internship or as a full-time career. Hospital chaplains are found both in secular and religious hospitals, administering to the spiritual needs of patients. In addition, members of the clergy from the community are generally welcome in any hospital or health care agency to minister to their parishioners or to any patient requesting a visit.

Hospitals generally employ at least one and sometimes many *professional record librarians* to oversee the compiling, filing, and storing of the patient records. Record librarians can be educated at the baccalaureate level. They have expertise in record keeping, conversion to computer software or to microfiche or microfilm forms, and storage and retrieval of information. Since accurate records are essential in providing continuity of care for patients, as well as protecting both consumer and provider legally, the role of the record librarian is crucial to the functioning of any health care institution.

A hospital or other health care agency with a library of any size will probably employ one or more professional *librarians*. A master's in library science is generally the entry level preparation for a professional librarian position. These persons are experts in the cataloging, ordering, maintenance, and resources provided by a library.

The category used by the Bureau of the Census entitled "health technologists and technicians" encompasses 1) persons prepared at the baccalaureate or higher degree level and 2) those with 1 to 2 years of preparation. This category includes laboratory technologists, x-ray technologists, radiotherapy technologists, and dental hygienists, as well as all persons known as technicians. Persons with a baccalaureate degree, such as laboratory technologists, generally are licensed professionals and supervise the work of technicians. The variety and number of such persons employed by a hospital or health care agency will vary, depending upon the services offered and the number of patients served. Laboratory, x-ray, and radiotherapy technologists have expertise in their specialties that includes the ability to make decisions about the manner in which a particular therapy or test is to be conducted, based on individual traits of their patients. For example, an x-ray technologist will position a patient for an x-ray based on the size, age, and sex of the patient, and the site of the injury or suspected disease. The laboratory technologist may oversee an entire laboratory under the direction of the pathologist or may have responsibility for a particular section, such as hematology or cytology.

Several other groups of professionals should be mentioned before we discuss paraprofessionals. These are individuals holding a master's or doctorate in public health whose expertise ranges from health care management (such as serving as the commissioner of health for a town, city, or state) to epidemiology, personpower, facilities, economics, quality and/ or organization of health care (Bowers & Purcell, 1974). In addition, there are persons holding degrees in psychology, anthropology, sociology, special education, and other disciplines who are employed in health care agencies and institutions as counselors, medical anthropologists, medical sociologists, educational evaluators, mental health care professionals, and other positions. These individuals may be involved in direct patient care through individual evaluation or in developing protocols for care and in policy and decision making.

Obviously, there are also many health care professionals who generally are in independent practice, such as dentists, podiatrists, homeopaths, osteopathic physicians, chiropractors, optometrists, and opticians. Sometimes these persons are employed by hospitals and other health care agencies.

Paraprofessionals

Paraprofessionals are, by definition, health care providers prepared at the associate degree or technical school level. They have special preparation in a particular field, such as respiratory therapy or x-ray technology, but work under the direct supervision and direction of a professional in their specialty area. They are hired directly by the institution and work as staff members in the department to which they are assigned.

Technicians

The variety of technicians employed in health care is evident in a list of schools offering programs to prepare technicians. Categories include: biomedical equipment, laboratory, dental, dietary, environmental, diagnostic (electroencephalograph, radiologic), inhalation, medical record, occupational and physical therapy, operating room, optician, prosthetic, mental health, and medical record technician (Kinsinger, 1970). In addition, medical secretaries and medical assistants constitute another group of persons who provide both direct care (such as taking a patient's history or temperature) and indirect care (typing and filing of medical records).

Support Service Personnel

The hospital employs many persons who are not responsible for direct care, but without whom care could not be given. These persons are employed in the physical plant and are responsible for the utilities, heat, cleaning, and maintenance of the building; for ordering, preparing, serving, and cleaning up for all food served; for communications throughout and outside of the hospital; for ordering, monitoring the use of, and disposing of all the supplies and equipment used; for transportation within the institution; and for all the laundry generated by staff and patients. There are people responsible for distributing televisions, flowers brought in by outside florists, mail, for taking photographs, for all hospital publications and forms used to keep records of patient stays, and for almost any function one can imagine in a business or home. In short, a hospital is, in a sense, a mini-community, and employs persons to do all the jobs one would find in a business or home setting.

Administrative Services

In order to keep this complex organization functioning, there have to be leaders or administrators. The structure of the administrative hierarchy varies from hospital to hospital, but there is generally a chief executive officer responsible for the day-to-day operations of several persons who share responsibility for the various subgroups within the institution. Each hospital has an organizational chart depicting the way in which the administration is set up, the lines of communication, and the place of nursing within the organization. Some examples appear in the appendix.

The variety of individuals employed within a hospital reflects the complexity of the organization. As the functions of hospitals grow more complex, more persons are necessary to provide both the direct and indirect services to patients that constitute hospital care. The person in the hospital will see many persons in the course of his or her hospitalization. The color and style of the clothing these people wear is no longer sufficient to let the patient know who the person is and what his or her role is to be. Thus it is particularly important that we identify ourselves to our patients as nurses and clearly explain our function in giving care.

Many of the persons discussed in this chapter also work or practice in community agencies. In the next chapter, we will discuss community health agencies and their role in providing care to consumers. It is probable that you will have some of your clinical experiences in the community, as the community, rather than the hospital, is the setting where most health care takes place.

REFERENCES

American Nurses' Association (1981). *Facts about nursing, '80–'81.* New York: American Journal of Nursing Company.

Bowers, J.Z. & Purcell, E.F. (1974). *Schools of public health: present and future.* New York: Josiah Macy Foundation.

Bullough, B. & Bullough, V.L. (1972). *Poverty, ethnic identity, and health care.* New York: Appleton-Century-Crofts.

Golden, A.S. (1979). The impact of new health professionals. In *Health care in the 1980s who provides? who plans? who pays?* New York: National League for Nursing, pp. 46–60.

Kinsinger, R.E., ed. (1970). *Health technicians.* Chicago: J.G. Ferguson.

Mason, M., Wenberg, B.G., & Welsh, P.K. (1982). *The dynamics of clinical dietetics,* 2nd ed. New York: John Wiley.

National League for Nursing (1982). *NLN nursing data book.* New York: National League for Nursing.

Resources Administration for Health Statistics (1976). *Health resources statistics 1975.* Rockville, Maryland: U.S. Department of Health, Education and Welfare, Public Health Service.

Statistical abstract of the United States 1984 (1984). Washington, D.C.: U.S. Department of Commerce, Bureau of the Census.

Statistical abstract of the United States 1985, 105th ed. Washington, D.C.: Bureau of the Census, U.S. Department of Commerce.

$$6$$

Health Agencies in the Community

Families and individuals are searching for alternatives in the health care delivery system. This search is sparked by the alarming spiraling of hospital costs, the arrival of Diagnosis Related Groups (DRGs), increasing consumer awareness of personal responsibility in health care, and a shift in focus from sickness care to health promotion and illness prevention.

This chapter addresses selected alternatives to hospital care. These alternatives include services rendered by official, voluntary, combination, hospital-based, and proprietary agencies in the community.

COMMUNITY HEALTH AGENCIES

Types of Health Agencies in the Community

The so-called "home health care agencies" in the community are many and varied. They all provide health care (to clients) that is in some way community- or home-based.

In general, their goal is to keep clients in the community. Many also have goals directed at keeping clients independent and healthy for as long as possible and/or supplementing the client's own abilities so that he/she can remain at home. Administrative and organizational structure provide a basis for identifying the five general types of home health care agencies (Stanhope and Lancaster, 1984). They are:

1. Official (public)
2. Unofficial (private and voluntary)
3. Combination
4. Hospital-based
5. Proprietary

While these types are not mutually exclusive, they do provide a framework in which to examine these agencies and their contribution to health care.

OFFICIAL AGENCIES

Official agencies, also known as public agencies, are operated by the state or by the local city and/or county government. These agencies, nonprofit entities, are heavily financed through the use of tax funds and are established by law to provide services to ensure maintenance of health of the public. In order to accomplish this mission, these agencies provide health education and disease prevention programs along with home care programs. A city health department is an example of an official agency.

In addition to this public funding, official agencies also receive money from other sources because they are sometimes reimbursed for services, as are other types of home care services. Private insurance companies, Blue Cross/Blue Shield, and Medicare and Medicaid provide full or partial reimbursement for some services through a complex payment

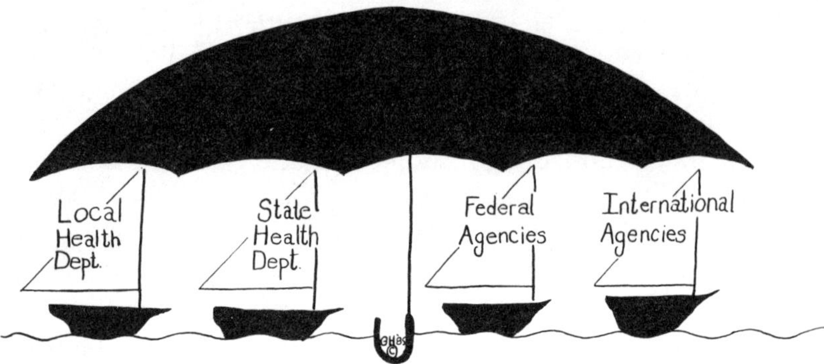

Figure 6.1 Types of Official Agencies. (© Glen D. Hawkins).

system. Due to these multiple funding sources, official agencies are frequently in a position to offer a fuller range of the health services to the community to meet their joint emphasis of health promotion and disease prevention than are private agencies.

Local

Because of a variety of factors, each local governmental health agency—whether it be town, city or county—varies in such areas as services offered and priorities. However, the agencies share some common responsibilities, functions, and structural features. For example, the local health department has three main responsibilities: 1) to assess its population's health status and needs, 2) to determine how well those needs are being met, and 3) to take action toward satisfying unmet needs (Hanlon and Pickett, 1984, p. 146).

The setting usually determines the structure of a local health department. A greater diversity and amount of work is required of a large metropolitan agency than of a small rural agency. In both instances, the local board of health has responsibility for the health of its citizens. Board members may be political appointees, be elected, or selected by officials or members of the community. The health officer, appointed by the board, usually employs the staff for the department. The health officer is usually a physician (40%) or has a B.S., B.A., M.A., or M.S., and most local health officers are male (74%). Two-thirds of the smallest departments are directed by women, usually nurses (Rohrer and Dellaportas, 1982).

The services and programs are similar for local and county health departments. These services are provided directly by employees of the health department or by contracts with other health care providers in the community, for example, the local Visiting Nurse Association. Five areas of service are addressed by official local health agencies. These areas are: 1) community health services, 2) environmental health services, 3) mental health services, 4) personal health services, and 5) processes common to all services. Table 6.1 identifies each of these areas and lists the specific services within each.

TABLE 6.1 Services of Local/County Health Departments[a]

Areas	Services
Community health	Facilities inspection and licensure Fire and housing inspection Health education Communicable disease control Immunizations
Environmental health	Milk and food inspection Rabies control Abate nuisances and filth Rat control and extermination services Water, sewage, waste disposal Radiation control Air pollution control Restaurant inspection and licensure
Mental health	Clinics Inpatient facilities Group homes Hotlines
Personal health	Pediatric, adult, older adult, ambulatory care School health

TABLE 6.1 *(Continued)*

	Dental health
	Neighborhood health centers
	Family planning
	Venereal disease care (VD)/sexually transmitted disease (STD)
	Tuberculosis (TB) care
	Home care
	Hospitals
	Screening for hypertension, glaucoma, diabetes
	Chronic disease care
	Care of indigent
	Occupational health
	Ambulance service
	Nutrition program
	Alcohol, drug programs
Processes common to all services	Laboratory services
	Record keeping
	Vital statistics, health statistics
	Health planning
	Rules and regulations
	Public health needs
	Resource assessment

[a] Source: Miller, C.A., Moos, M.K., Kotch, J.B., Brown, M.B. and Brainard, M.P. *American Journal of Public Health,* 1981; 71(Supplement):15–29.

Chang, A. *American Journal of Public Health,* 1981; 71:31–33.

Miller, C.A., Brooks, E.F., DeFriese, G.H., Gilbert, B., Jain, S.C., and Kavaler, F. *American Journal of Public Health* 1977; 67(10):931–939.

Many people utilize services provided by the local health departments. Each year about 40% of the people receive some personal health service; 50% of poverty-stricken children utilize services of public agencies for part or all of their medical care (Miller, et al., 1981).

Just as the setting of the health department may vary, so may the personnel employed. However, a common cadre of personnel will usually be found in most agencies, all working toward the prevention of disease and promotion of health. These personnel, in addition to the health officer, include: staff physician, public health nurses, public health laboratory technician, dentist, sanitarians, industrial hygienist, statistician, chemist, health educator, and social workers (Smolensky, 1977). Personnel may provide direct care or serve as educators or consultants (Figure 6.2).

State

Each of the 50 state health departments in the United States provides the following services:

1. seeking the causes of communicable disease in man and domestic animals
2. investigation of the sources of morbidity and mortality
3. investigation of the effects of localities, employment conditions, and circumstances on public health
4. licensing of hospitals and nursing homes
5. detection and prevention of adulteration of food and drugs
6. examination for and the prevention of pollution of public water and ice supplies
7. preparation and distribution, at cost, or antitoxins, vaccines, and other approved biologic products for the control or prevention of communicable diseases. (Smolensky, 1977)

The internal structure is designed by each state to meet the various regulations and needs of the population. The state provided services are most apt to be educational and supportive rather than in the provision of direct care. Services that may be included are listed in Table 6.2.

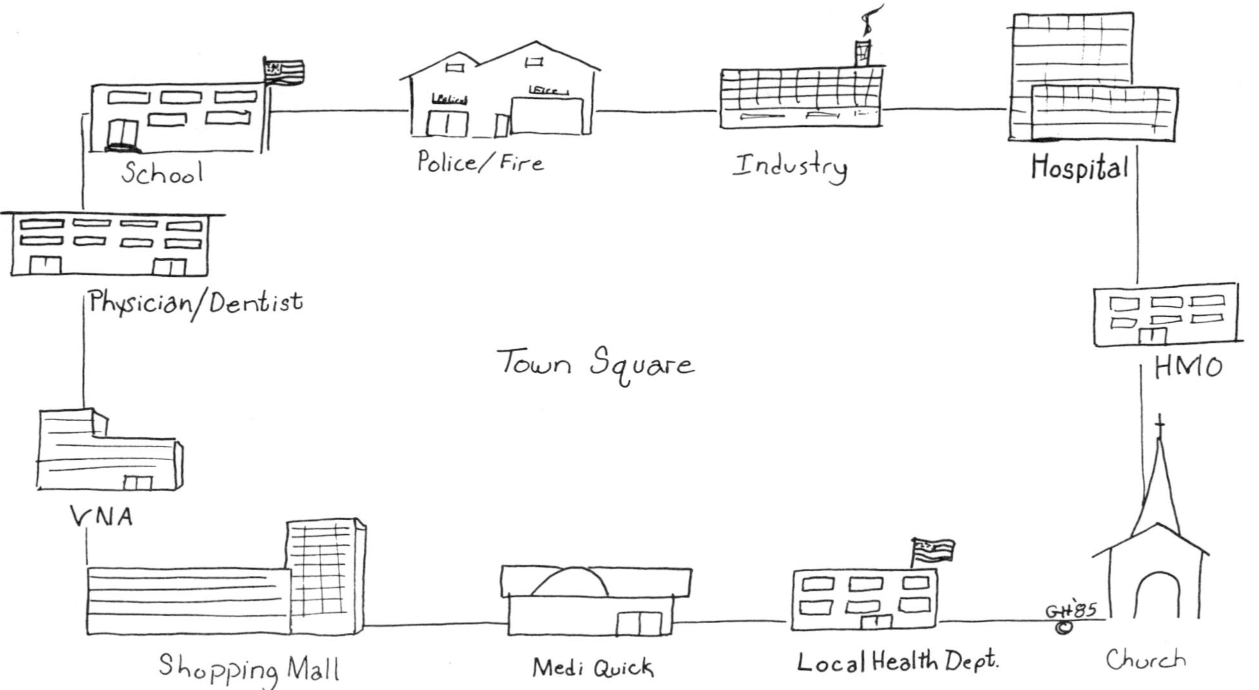

Figure 6.2 Health care agencies in the community. (© Glen D. Hawkins).

TABLE 6.2 State Health Department Functions[a]

Services Commonly Provided
Immunization programs
Environmental surveillance
Tuberculosis control
Maternal–child health
School health program
Venereal disease control
Chronic disease programs
Home care
Family planning
Ambulatory care
Mental health

[a]Source: Miller, C.A., Brooks, E.F., DeFriese, G.H., Gilbert, B., Jain, S.C., and Kavaler, F. *American Journal of Public Health* 1977; 67(10):931–939.

Federal

The *federal* level is the most complex level of the health care system. The Department of Health and Human Services (DHHS) is the umbrella cabinet-level department for most agencies concerned with health. The Public Health Service (PHS), directed by the Surgeon General, is one unit in this department (DHHS) and encompasses the Centers for Disease Control (CDC); the Food and Drug Administration (FDA); the National Institutes of Health (NIH); the Alcohol, Drug Abuse, and Mental Health Administration; and the Health Resources and Services Administration (HRSA). Administration of grants and contracts is the major function of each of these component agencies, as well as protecting and providing for the health of the public through policy making, overseeing of policy enforcement, collection of vital and health statistics, planning for research for present and future needs, and some direct provision of care (Hawkins and Higgins, 1985).

The Division of Nursing is part of the Bureau of Health Professions, in turn part of the Health Resources and Services Administration (HRSA) of the United States Public Health Service (PHS), Department of Health and Human Services (DHHS). The Division of Nursing staff members attempt to increase the quality and availability of health services by promoting the role of nurses in health care delivery. The Division supports research and education in nursing and reviews nursing issues, prepares literature about nursing, and is a clearinghouse for information about nursing (Division of Nursing, undated).

International

We do not live in isolation. Therefore, our international neighbors are very important to us in many ways; and health is no exception. The World Health Organization (WHO) of the United Nations serves "as the one directing and coordinating authority on international health work" (Hanlon and Pickett, 1984, p. 79). Examples of other international organizations include Pan American Health Organization and the United Nations Children's Fund. These organizations all try to coordinate health related activities and to explore issues of common concern, as well as to plan jointly for solutions to common problems.

In summary, there are official agencies organized at the local, state, federal, and international levels. Through a complex system of delivery, both direct and supportive services are rendered to the various populations served. Understanding our place in the complex supersystem helps in coping with the levels of bureaucracy with which we must at times deal.

PRIVATE AND VOLUNTARY AGENCIES

Private and voluntary agencies provide health services to groups of people on a *voluntary* basis; that is to say that they are not *required* by law to do this. Funding is through a variety of sources including: private contributions, philanthropic gifts, charities, and fund raising, and some third-party monies (primarily Medicare and Medicaid, but also private insurance companies and Blue Cross/Blue Shield). The financial resources available depend, to a large extent, on the community served. The visiting nurse associations have been the classic examples of this type of health agency. The Visiting Nurse Association of Chicago was founded in 1889. Its first home was in Hull House and Jane Addams was a charter member (VNA, 1979). In 1893, Lillian Wald and Mary Brewster started a visiting nurse service for the poor people in New York. This led to the development of the Henry Street Settlement (Wald, 1915). The Henry Street Settlement is an important example of a neighborhood house that offered to the community a variety of social, recreational, educational, and health services. Community members could come to Henry Street to attend classes on a variety of topics, to discuss problems in their homes such as lack of heat or sanitary facilities, to enjoy social events such as dances, and to use the services of the visiting nurses.

Voluntary and private nonprofit agencies are exempt from federal income tax and are nongovernmental agencies. Traditionally, the client's need for a given service was the basis for provision of service. Financial exigency has had an impact on this method of allocation of services by the voluntary agencies. These agencies are typically governed by lay boards of directors, serving on a voluntary basis, and representative of the community served. The agencies are privately held entities, generally incorporated.

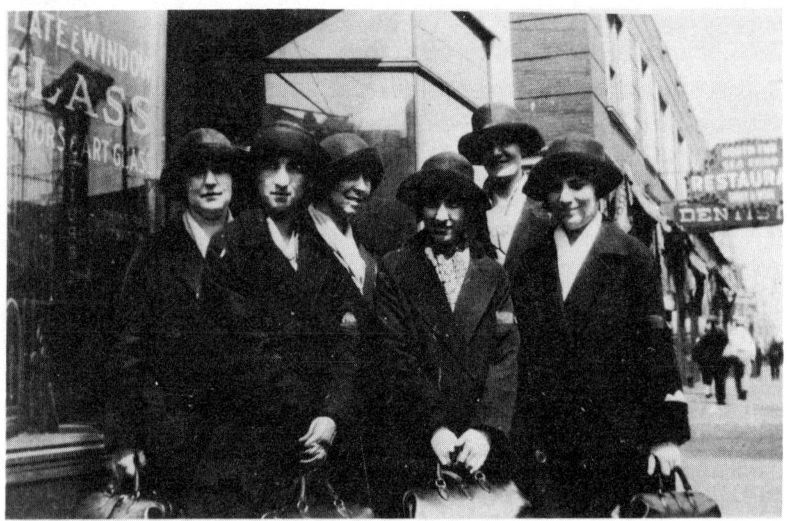

Figure 6.3 Visiting Nurses: VNA of Chicago in the 1920s.

Since 1892—with the establishment of the Anti-Tuberculosis Society as the first voluntary health group—100,000 voluntary health/disease agencies have been formed (Hanlon & Pickett, 1984).

According to Hanlon and Pickett (1984, p. 160), voluntary agencies have made contributions to health care by:

1. Pioneering and trying out new ideas and methods
2. Demonstrating a variety of techniques to improve health
3. Providing health education functions, including client, public, and professional training
4. Supplementation of official activities
5. Guarding citizens' interests in health by being watchdogs of what is being developed in their areas
6. Promoting health legislation
7. Developing well-balanced community health programs by filling in the gaps left by the service restrictions of other agencies
8. Planning and coordination

Voluntary agencies are frequently one of four types (Hanlon and Pickett, 1984, p. 159): 1) agencies concerned with specific diseases, such as the American Diabetic Society and the American Cancer Society; 2) agencies concerned with certain structures or organs of the body, such as The American Society for the Hard of Hearing and the National Society for Crippled Children; 3) agencies concerned with the health and welfare of special groups in society, such as the Maternity Association of New York; and 4) agencies concerned with particular phases of health and welfare, for example, Planned Parenthood Federation of America. The list of agencies within each grouping goes on and on. Complete lists can be found in reference works in most libraries.

Private foundations, such as W. K. Kellogg and Robert Wood Johnson, and professional associations such as the American Nurses Association, American Medical Association, and the National League for Nursing are also voluntary and generally nonprofit agencies. The private foundations (R.W. Johnson, Kellogg) generally support research and/or delivery of health services to special groups and also are sometimes involved in the education of health care professionals. Directories of private foundations are available in community and university libraries (Foundation Directory, 1985).

Professional organizations exist primarily to serve their members, to set standards for practice, and to advance the profession for the public good. A complete list of professional nursing organizations is published annually in the *American Journal of Nursing* (*AJN,* 1985).

Although you will undoubtedly have contact with many community-based voluntary agencies concerned with health in your career, you are likely to have some experience as a student in a Visiting Nurse Association (VNA). As you will recall, the VNA is the classic example of a voluntary agency. The VNA, a multifaceted agency, provides a variety of home health care services tailored to meet individual needs. Naturally, each agency is unique. However, there are certain services commonly offered by VNAs. These services fall into the broad categories of nursing; therapy; homemaker/home health aid; and medical social work. Within each of these categories are specific services. For example, nursing services may include skilled nursing care; chemotherapy; intravenous therapy; nutrition; health screening; and health counseling. Physical, occupational, and speech therapy are covered under the category "therapy." Homemaker/home health aid services include personal care, housekeeping, and meal preparation. Medical social work coordinates community services; provides counseling, social, and financial evaluations; and agencies and community services provide information about and referral to these as appropriate.

The staffing of such an agency must be appropriate for the services it renders. Staffing would be determined by the number and variety of goals to be met. Typically, the following professional staff members are active in VNAs: public health nurses, dieticians, physical therapists, occupational therapists, speech therapists, social workers, psychologists, and a whole cadre of assistants in the homemaker and home health aid service. Some services are provided by agency personnel, and other services (such as speech therapy) may be provided by a contract with the agency.

Visiting nurse associations or services (a VNA is sometimes a VNS) are generally guided by a board of directors, volunteers from the community, and funded through a combination of third-party reimbursement for services (Medicaid, Medicare, private insurance, and Blue Cross/Blue Shield), fee-for-service paid by clients, and money donated by or raised by members of the board of directors and the community at large. Sometimes a VNA will also contract with the town or county to provide certain services and, therefore, be paid out of public funds.

Due to diminishing private resources, competition from proprietary agencies (to be discussed later in this chapter) and shifts in services for which reimbursement by third party is available, many small VNAs are combining to serve a larger geographic area. For example, in one New England state, five VNAs merged to serve a five town area and yet three others merged to serve those three communities. Duplication of services and of support systems such as secretaries, office space, and so on is thus eliminated. Of course, certain costs, such as transportation to a wider area, must be considered in such mergers, as well as any stipulations made by the founding or endowing members of such agencies.

Hospice and the Health Maintenance Organization (HMO) are both settings for the delivery of health care in the community. Generally both are considered in the voluntary agency realm and are therefore briefly described in this section. As HMOs become more numerous, however, it should be noted that some have been established by groups of private investors, insurance companies, and corporations as profit-making enterprises.

Hospices

The term Hospice originally meant a medieval guest house or way station for travelers. During the time of the Crusades, hospices provided refuge for pilgrims on their way to and from the Holy Land. Currently the term hospice has come to be associated with a philosophy of care for persons in the last stages of life and for their families, and/or significant others. Hospices of the 20th century in England are freestanding facilities not associated with hospitals. These facilities are autonomous in terms of professional procedures and were the predecessors of the hospice movement in the United States.

There are several models of *hospice care* in the United States. Examples of these models include: an organization sponsored by a community home health agency; an acute care hospital model; an independent hospice program; an all-volunteer hospice; or a case management hospice model.

Through the Division of Nursing (USPHS), a comprehensive guide for development of a hospice and for staff and volunteer education has been developed. (See *Hospice Education for Nurses*).

Hospice is a caring community of professional and non-professional staff, augmented by a vast array of volunteer services. Patients who are not expected to live more than several months and are not receiving treatment to attempt cure of their diseases can be admitted to hospice services.

Hospice care offers comprehensive (both palliative and supportive) home care services for terminally ill patients and their families. Emotional, spiritual, and medical problems are addressed with a focus on the control of pain and other symptoms, maintaining the patient at home at an optimum level of functioning. Inpatient care is usually available when care of the patient at home becomes unmanageable for the family.

Care is provided by an interdisciplinary team. Members of this team will vary with the setting, but may include nurses, physicians, social workers, clergy, dieticians, home health aids, homemakers, and volunteers. Hospice staff members provide support to the family throughout their period of bereavement after the patient dies. By decreasing the amount of time patients spend in high cost hospital facilities, hospice has also proven to be a cost-effective model for health care delivery.

Health Maintenance Organizations

Health Maintenance Organizations (HMOs) first developed about the turn of the 19th century and were initially called prepaid group practices. They developed as a result of the westward movement that was made possible by the railroads and the industrial development that followed.The first HMO was the Kaiser Permanente Health Plan, designed to attract workers for shipbuilding operations during World War II. Today this plan is the largest HMO in the United States, covering nine geographic areas, with a membership of 4.6 million (Mayer, 1985, p. 592).

Over the past 10–15 years there has been rapid growth in the HMO movement. Dr. Paul Ellwood, a leader of this movement, concluded that "the existing fee-for-service system created 'perverse incentives', which rewarded physicians and institutions for treating illness and then withdrew those rewards when health was restored" (Mayer, 1985, p. 593). Thereby, preventive care was not valued.

As defined in 1971 by the then Department of Health, Education and Welfare (DHEW) (later changed to (DHHS), an HMO is an organized system of health care that assures delivery of an agreed upon set of comprehensive health maintenance, preventive, and treatment services for a voluntarily enrolled group within a geographic area. Services rendered are financed by the pre-negotiated and fixed periodic payment of the membership (Jonas, 1981). The HMO concept has gradually gained federal backing. The Health Maintenance Organization Act of 1973 (P.L. 93–222) set the requirement that all companies employing at least 25 persons must offer them the opportunity to have health insurance or membership in an HMO, if available. Additional legislation provided funds for the development and expansion of HMOs. The HMO Act of 1973 defined the organizational structure, basic and supplemental services, and basis for determining rate of prepayment (National League for Nursing, 1978, p.2). The amendment in 1976 required consumers to be involved in decision-making, and all HMOs receiving Medicare and Medicaid funds were to have federal qualification and regulation. The HMO amendments of 1978 added loan programs, programs for training HMO administrators and other management personnel, and provisions for technical assistance for HMO development. The amendments of 1981 increased flexibility in the organization of the HMOs and concern with the fiscal integrity (Wilson and Neuhauser, 1982, p. 211).

The National League for Nursing notes the following five characteristics of HMOs:

1. Organization makes a contract with consumers (or employers on their behalf) to assure the delivery of stated health services.
2. Benefits are comprehensive and include physicians' services, hospital care, ambulatory care, and preventive care.
3. Voluntarily enrolled population, sometimes referred to as a defined population.
4. Prepayment; that is, the HMO receives a payment in advance from each enrolled participant.
5. Emphasis on preventive medicine, keeping the patient well through primary care services.

Naturally, each HMO is unique. The services and coverage will vary. However, it is a general rule of thumb for HMOs that all medical services received by members of a given HMO must be rendered or authorized by an HMO physician. Table 6.3 lists services provided by one HMO and is reflective of the services offered by most of the HMOs.

Some services are, in general, not covered by HMOs. These services include: custodial care, blood or blood plasma; per-

TABLE 6.3 Services Generally Provided by HMO[a]

All visits to HMO physicians and other health care providers
Periodic physical examinations, including immunizations, routine gyne-
    cological care, hearing, and vision examinations
Routine well-child care
X-ray, laboratory, EKG, and other diagnostic services
Allergy tests and treatments
Pre- and postnatal care for woman and infant
Minor surgery
Medication, casts, and dressings
Mental health care for short-term evaluation or crisis intervention (des-
    ignated number of visits per year)
Health education
Prescription drugs (may be a small fee such as $1/prescription)
Room and board for semiprivate hospital room
All other medically necessary services
Physician's services
Surgeon's services
Anesthesia
Maternity care, including services required due to complications in delivery
Newborn care
Drugs/medications
X-ray, laboratory services
Private-duty nursing
Therapy, including radiation, inhalation, and chemotherapy
Administration of blood
Care (up to 120 days) for mental or nervous disorders
Home health services deemed medically necessary
Emergency care for life-threatening situations
Care for emergency illness or accidental injury
Ambulance service when medically necessary
Prosthetics (devices replacing body parts . . . excludes dental prosthetics)
Durable equipment (wheelchairs, hospital beds, etc.)
Orthopedic braces
Care in approved extended care facility
Specialized treatment for alcohol and drug abuse (limited coverage; des-
    ignated number of visits per year and during lifetime)

[a] Adapted from: "Now There's A New Way To Care, The HMO of
Delaware."

sonal comfort items; plastic or cosmetic surgery; military-
related disabilities; dental care, except for removal of bony
impacted teeth; experimental procedures; hearing aids; eye-

glasses or contact lenses; and any service not deemed medically necessary by the HMO physician. While many of the advantages of an HMO are evident, a limited choice or no choice of facilities is frequently cited as a deterrent to HMO membership.

Personnel with the background and in numbers necessary to provide the identified services are employed at the HMOs. These personnel typically include: physicians, nurses, nurse practitioners, nurse midwives, health educators, pharmacists, lab technicians, x-ray technicians, physicians' assistants, and numerous support service personnel.

HMOs, numbering about 323, currently serve 15 million members. Thirty-seven of the nation's 38 major metropolitan areas have at least one HMO (Mayer, 1985, p. 394). The Health Maintenance Organization movement continues to grow today as more individuals select this option for personal/family health care delivery.

COMBINATION AGENCIES

Combination agencies, as the name implies, refers to the merging of two types of agencies: typically, a voluntary and an official agency have joined to provide health care. In this way the agencies can maximize their resources by eliminating duplication of services and decreasing costs while maintaining services. An example of a combination agency is a VNA which also contracts with the town or city in which it is located to provide the home care and public health nursing needs of that community. Some communities are too small or too sparsely populated to justify 1) both having a VNA and 2) hiring public health nurses to perform health department nursing functions; therefore, a combination agency is a viable alternative.

HOSPITAL-BASED AGENCIES

These agencies are located in, adjacent to, or under the auspices of hospitals and their structure, and depend on the specific "parent" hospital structure. The board of directors of the hospital is responsible for the governance of the agency. These agencies can be of any of the organizational structures—official, voluntary, private, nonprofit—congruent with the structure of the hospital. A major advantage of these agencies is access and availability of all the hospital services. Over 250 hospitals located across the United States have some form of hospital-administered home care programs. Basic services provided include discharge care and coordination of care at home with other community-based agencies.

PROPRIETARY AGENCIES

Proprietary agencies are profit making agencies, and as such are not eligible for tax exemption status. The owner(s) receive all the profits from the income. Governance is the responsibility of the owner, and varies from an individual to a business corporation with a board of directors; and stock is 1) held in total privately or 2) traded in the open market. Reimbursement for services is primarily by clients and third-party payers, depending on the licensing laws of the state and the approval status of the given agency (e.g., eligibility for Medicare and Medicaid reimbursement). Specifically, an agency or a state with licensing laws and meeting all the standards can be licensed and approved to receive Medicare reimbursement for specific services.

Home health care personnel employed by proprietary agencies are reflective of the services the agency provides. Generally, personnel include: registered nurses; licensed practical nurses; speech, occupational, and physical therapists; home health aides; nurse assistants; companions; and homemakers.

The number of proprietary agencies is increasing. An example of this type of agency is Upjohn Health Care Services, with a 90-year history of high quality care. Upjohn has a philosophy of nursing services, objectives of care, and home health care clients' bill of rights.

Critics of proprietary agencies are worried that the profit motive—rather than concern for the well-being of clients—will drive the agency. There is also concern about rendering of substandard care by the nonlicensed agencies. Another aspect of the issue is that the nonregulated agencies might have more freedom in addressing specific client needs/requests. Of note is the lack of valid evidence that one type of agency provides a different—either higher or lower—quality of care than another (Home Health Line, 1976).

Most communities have a variety of services, agencies, and home health care programs. To assist in finding the best programs for your needs or the needs of clients, several suggestions can be offered. The family physician and social service director of the local hospital are likely to know appropriate community resources. Other sources are organizations such as the Visiting Nurses' Association; yellow pages of the telephone directory under several headings, including health care services; and the director of city, county, or state Public Health Services/the Office of the United States Public Health Service/the Administrator of a Veterans' Administration Hospital.

In summary, this chapter addressed official, voluntary, combination, hospital-based, and proprietary health agencies in the community which are reflective of the diversity and complexity of the health care delivery system. Knowing about the agencies and services available is necessary for both consumers and providers of health care so that informed choices can be made.

REFERENCES

1985 Directory of Nursing Organizations. *American Journal of Nursing* 1985;8(4):493–496, 498, 500.

American Journal of Public Health 1981;71(1) (Supplement): whole issue. Role of state and local governments in relation to personal health services.

Chang, A. (1981). Primary health care for urban children and youth: the role of local health departments. *American Journal of Public Health,* 71(1)(Supplement):31–33.

Division of Nursing. U.S. Department of Health and Human Services, PHS, HRSA, Bureau of Health Professions.

Division of Nursing, USPHS, DHHS. *Hospice Education for Nurses.* Copies available from the U.S. Department of Commerce, National Technical Information Service, 52895 Port Royal Road, Springfield, VA 22161. (Pub #HRP 0904175.)

Hanlon, J.J., and Pickett, C.E. (1984). *Public Health: Administration and Practice,* 8th ed. St. Louis: C.V. Mosby.

Hawkins, J.W., and Higgins, L.P. (1985). *Nursing and American Health Care System,* 2nd ed. New York: Tiresias Press.

Home Health Line (1976). 1(13):88.

Jonas, S. (1981). Ambulatory care. In S. Jonas (ed.) *Health Care Delivery in the United States.* New York: Springer, pp. 126–168.

Mayer, T.R. (1985). HMOs: origins and development. *The New England Journal of Medicine,* 312(9):590–594.

Miller, C.A., Brooks, E.F., DeFriese, G.H., Gilbert, B., Jain, S.C., and Kavaler, F. (1977). A survey of local public health departments and their directors. *American Journal of Public Health,* 67(10):931–939.

Miller, C.A., Moos, M.K., Kotch, J.B., Brown, M.B., and Brainard, M.P. (1981). The role of local health departments in the delivery of ambulatory care. *American Journal of Public Health,* 71(Supplement):15–29.

National League for Nursing (1978). Health Maintenance Organization.

Rohrer, H.H., Dellaportas, G. (1982). Trends and patterns in characterstics of local health administrators. *American Journal of Public Health* 1982, 72(8):846–849.

Smolensky, J. (1977). *Principles of Community Health,* 4th ed. Philadelphia: W. B. Saunders.

Stanhope, M., Lancaster, J. (1984). *Community Health Nursing: Process and Practice for Promoting Health.* St. Louis: C.V. Mosby.

The Foundation Center. *Foundation Directory* (1983). New York.

Visiting Nurse Association (1979). *90th Annual Report.* Chicago.

Wald, L.D. (1915). *The House on Henry Street.* New York: Henry Holt and Company.

Wilson, F.A., Neuhauser, D. (1982). *Health Services in the United States.* Cambridge, MA: Ballinger Publishing Company.

Appendix A

A Comparison of Blue Cross/ Blue Shield and Commercial Health Insurance[a]

Blue Cross/Blue Shield	Commercial Health Insurance
Health insurance their only business	Some—health insurance is only business; most—part of life or casualty insurance companies
Payment directly to the provider group, such as physician or hospital group experience rated—rate for coverage based on the group to be covered	Cash payment to the insured; sometimes payment to provider; experience rated—rates based on the previous experience of the company
Deals directly with physicians and hospitals—pays provider	Generally deals with the insured person, although some companies will now pay the provider

Blue Cross/Blue Shield	Commercial Health Insurance
Nonprofit	Established for profit
Some deductibles—patient pays the first $_____ of the bill	Some deductibles
Coinsurance—plan may pay 80% of a single room	Coinsurance
Limitations on coverage—plan pays for so many days of hospital care in a given year; pays for certain tests but not for others, etc.	Limitations on coverage
Group and individual plans—one can join as part of a group such as through one's place of employment as a benefit or as an individual (fees are significantly different)	Group and individual plans
Blue Cross: hospitalization insurance; Blue Shield: in-hospital physician services, limited office visits, some dental care, prescription drugs, some home health care, nursing home care	Hospitalization insurance; in-hospital physician services; limited office visits; some dental, home health care, prescription drugs
Some group major medical policies	Major medical policies; some cash payment policies (cash payments directly to insured)

Blue Cross/Blue Shield	Commercial Health Insurance
Rates supervised and monitored by the state insurance commissioner	Supervised by state insurance commissioner; no rate regulation except that rates be high enough to cover claims
Benefits generally measure in units of service, such as so many days in hospital, so many physician visits	Benefits measured in cash amounts
Company can invest premium money	Company can invest premium money
Insure <50% of Americans who have insurance	Insure >50% of Americans who have insurance
67 Blue Cross, 68 Blue Shield Plans	More than 1,000 commercial companies
Strive for success of member hospitals and physicians	Strive to generate a surplus in order to pay dividends to their shareholders
Board of directors dominated by hospital representatives	Boards of directors—founders of the companies or representatives of their interests

[a]Synthesized from many sources, including: 1) *Blue Cross/Blue Shield Fact Book 1981* (1981), Chicago: Blue Cross/Blue Shield; 2) Hetherington, R.W., Hopkins, C.E. & Roemer, M.I. (1975), *Health insurance plans: promise and performance,* New York: Wiley; 3) Jacobs, P. (1980), *The economics of health and medical care,* Baltimore: University Park Press; 4) Law, S.A. (1974), *Blue Cross what went wrong?,* New Haven: Yale University Press; 5) *Source book of health insurance data 1981–1982* (1982), Washington, D.C.: Health Insurance Association of America.

Appendix B

A Comparison of Medicare and Medicaid[a]

Medicare	Medicaid
Amendment to Social Security Act 1965, Title 18	Amendment to Social Security Act 1965, Title 19
Hospital insurance for the aged and those with permanent disabilities	Grants to states for medical assistance programs for those eligible for the aid under the state's eligibility criteria
Administered at the federal level—Social Security Administration	Administered at federal, state, and local levels (50 different programs)
Financed by % payroll tax paid by employees and employer under FICA and deducted directly from pay	Financed by cost sharing between federal government and each state

Medicare	Medicaid
Eligibility—all persons 65 and older	Eligibility varies from state to state: includes institutionalized elders, poor elders, those eligible for Aid to Families with Dependent Children (known as "welfare"); Supplemental Security Income for the blind; individuals who have disabilities or are medically indigent; often leave out many persons without the means to seek health care
Part A: hospitalization (paid for by the FICA payroll deduction tax) Part B: physician's services; to enroll in this there is a monthly premium to be paid by the insured person	
Coverage mandated by the federal government; now under a prospective payment plan whereby the fee for service for a hospital stay is based on DRGs (diagnosis related groups) that allocate so many days of hospital care for a particular condition and then the person must be discharged	Certain services mandated by federal government; program design and benefits left to the individual states; hospital care will have same prospective payment scheme as Medicare

Medicare	Medicaid
25 million persons eligible and number is growing as population ages	24 million persons eligible and number may shrink as the eligibility criteria as to income are more stringent
Pays less than 50% of the health bills of older adults	Estimates of up to 5–13% of persons in this country with no health insurance and not eligible for Medicaid
Major expenditures for hospitalization	Major expenditures for nursing home and intermediate care facilities, then hospital care
Coinsurance and deductibles	Virtually no coinsurance, but benefits vary considerably from state to state
Free choice of provider	Must use provider who will accept Medicaid patients

[a]References include: Williams, C.A., ed. (1984), *Nursing research and policy formation: the case of prospective payment.* Kansas City, Missouri: American Academy of Nursing.

Appendix C
Selected Health Care Resources in the Community[a]

Al-Anon
Alcoholics Anonymous
American Cancer Society
American Diabetes
  Association
American Heart Association
American Red Cross
Arthritis Foundation
Association for the Blind
Association for Retarded
  Citizens
Big Brothers–Big Sisters
Birthright
Childbirth and Parenting
  Education Association
Children's Bureau
Crippled Children and
  Adults Society
Crisis Pregnancy Center
Deaf Contact
Food Bank

Genetic Services
Home Health Care
Information and Referral
  Service
Juvenile Diabetes
  Foundation
Leukemia Society of
  America
March of Dimes Birth
  Defects Foundation
Multiple Sclerosis National
  Society
National Kidney Foundation
Parents Anonymous
Planned Parenthood
Rape Crisis Center
Red Cross
Rehabilitation Center
State Health Council
State Lung Association
United Cerebral Palsy

[a] This listing is not all inclusive. It is representative of the variety of agencies and groups in a medium sized city. Please consult your local telephone directory for additional resources and the needed telephone numbers and addresses.

Appendix D Department of Nursing Organizational Chart

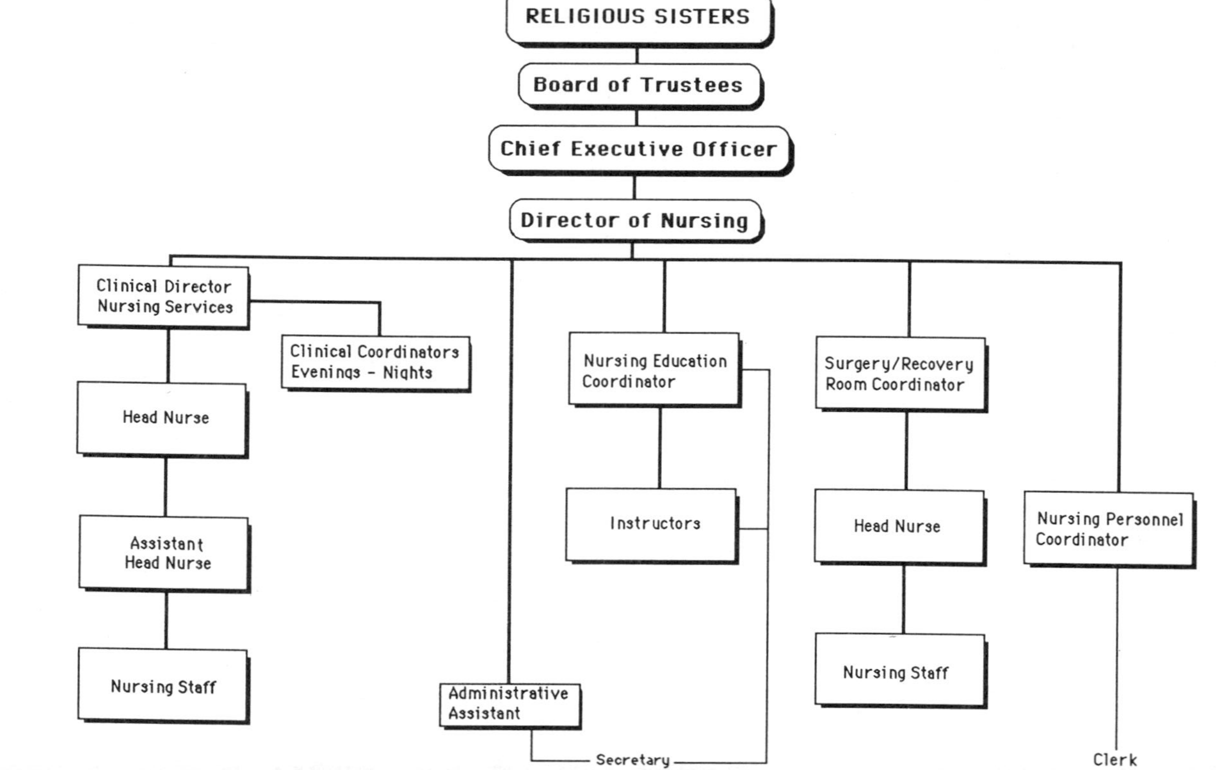

Appendix E Nursing Service Organizational Chart

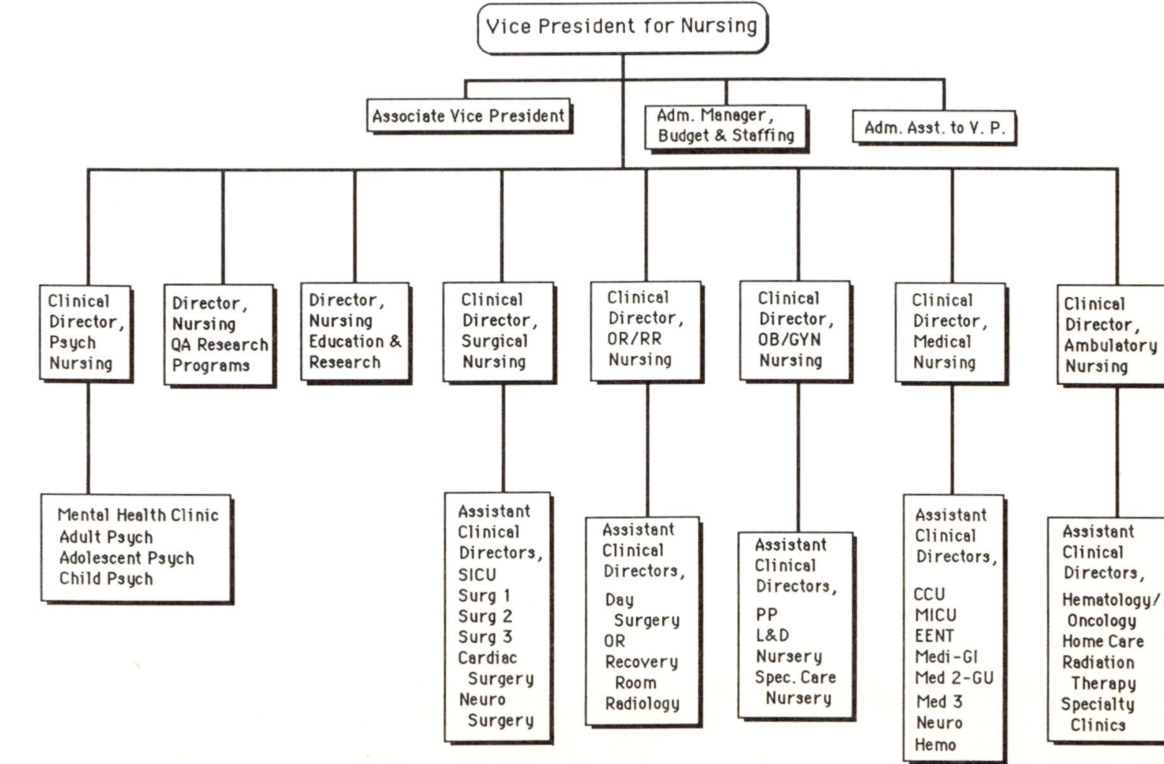

Glossary

AC/PC—before and after meals
ADL—activities of daily living
Ad. Lib.—as much as desired
Alopecia—hair loss or baldness
Amb.—ambulatory
Ambulate—to walk
ASHD—arteriosclerotic heart disease
BID—twice a day
BM—bowel movement
Board of Health—a group of people usually headed by the local health officer. May be appointed or elected and are concerned with administration of the laws concerning health.
BP—blood pressure
BRP—bathroom privileges
BUN—blood urea nitrogen
c̄—with

C—celsius or centigrade
CA—cancer
Cal—calorie
CAT scanner—computerized axial tomography
Cath—catheterization
C & B—chair and blanket; means patient may be up and sit in the chair
CBC—complete blood count
CC—cubic centimeter
CCU—coronary care unit
Communicable Disease—an infectious disease that may be transmitted from one source (either animal or person) to another directly or indirectly (such as a vector).
Community—a group of individuals/families living in a given area having a united

interest or membership in a given organization.

Community Health—This is the goal of community oriented practice, management and meeting of collective health needs.

Consultant—one who gives professional advice and services; one considered to have expertise. A consulting health care worker (nurse, physician, pharmacist) who shares expertise in advisory capacity.

Cost Effectiveness—the relationship of an item, program, or service to the cost of the identified goal or outcome

C/S—culture and sensitivity

CT Scan—CAT scan or computerized axial tomography

CVA—cerebral vascular accident; stroke

CVS—clean voided specimen

DC—discontinue or discharge

D & C—dilatation and curretage (of cervix and uterus)

Department of Health—an organization that protects and regulates the health of the people in its constituency at the local, state or federal level

Disease Prevention—activities and services that are designed to avoid threats to health; examples are clean air standards, immunizations

DTV—due to void

Dx—diagnosis

EEG—electroencephalogram

EENT—eye, ear, nose, and throat

ENT—ear, nose, and throat

EKG or ECG—electrocardiogram

Emesis—vomitus

Endoscopy—looking into an organ or cavity

Environment—all the conditions that surround and influence living things

ER—emergency room

F—fahrenheit

FBS—fasting blood sugar

Federal Register—published by the U.S. government every working day detailing regulations, changes, challenge periods and meeting schedules of the many offices, departments and agencies of the federal government

Fee-for-Service—the payment system in which the charge is based on the particular service rendered

Fx—fracture

GI—gastrointestinal

GTT—glucose tolerance test

Guaiac—test for occult blood

Health—well-being; of sound mind and body; environment

and individual (organism) in dynamic equilibrium to maintain integrity of optimal functioning

Health Care—the result of services (preventive, remedial, and therapeutic) directed at preventing and treating diseases and promoting a maximum level of functioning in individuals and groups

Health Consumer—one who uses health services

Health Education—service directed to the general public to foster adoption of a life style that promotes healthful living

Health Maintenance Organization—a prepaid health care program; services focus on health promotion and education; comprehensive medical care is available

Health Promotion—a combination of activities to facilitate the attainment of optimal level of wellness of an individual, family, or group (community or organization)

Health Provider—one who performs health services such as a nurse or physician

HMO—health maintenance organization

HN—head nurse

Hospice—an interdisciplinary program for the care of the terminally ill and their families in the home or hospital setting; provides supportive and palliative care with the primary concern of relief of symptoms (e.g., pain, nausea) and maximum level of comfort and well-being

ICU—intensive care unit

ID—intradermal

IM—intramuscular

Industrial Hygienist—a member of the occupational health team with expertise in several areas including air analysis, monitoring techniques and standards set by the Occupational Safety and Health Administration (OSHA) of the federal government

I & O—intake and output

IPPB—intermittent positive pressure breathing devices

IV—intravenously

Johnny—a patient hospital gown

Lab—laboratory where tests are done

L & D—labor and delivery

LPN—licensed practical nurse

LVN—licensed vocational nurse

Mammogram—x-ray of the breasts

Mat—maternity

MD—medical doctor; physician

Medicaid—program jointly funded by the state and federal government to provide access to medical care for the poor; those without health insurance

Medicare—hospitalization insurance for older adults

Meds—medications

Mental Health—implies positive adaptation to the environment as demonstrated by satisfaction from one's interpersonal relationships; ability to cope with every day stressors

Metastasis—spreading of cancer or tumor cells

MI—myocardial infarction; heart attack

MICU—medical intensive care unit

NA—nursing aide or assistant

Neoplasm—malignant tumor

Neuro—neurology

NICU—neonatal intensive care unit

Noc—night

Nonprofit—not for profit; implies an altruistic motive

NPO—nothing by mouth

O$_2$—oxygen

OB—obstetrics

Oncology—diagnosis and treatment of tumors or cancer

OOB—out of bed

OPD—outpatient department

OR—operating room

Ortho—orthopedics

OT—occupational therapy

P̄—after

P—pulse

Path—pathology

Pedi—pediatrics

Peds—pediatrics

PH—public health

Pharm—pharmacy

PICU—pediatric intensive care unit

Proprietary—operated for profit

Per—through or by

PO—by mouth (*per os*)

Postop—postoperative

PP—postpartum

Preop—preoperative

Prepaid Coverage—payment system in which the individual/family pays a set amount for a given time period for comprehensive health care coverage regardless of the services actually used; an HMO is an example

PRN—whenever necessary

PT—physical therapy

QD—daily; every day

QID—four times a day

QS—quantities sufficient

R—respirations

RBC—red blood count

RD—registered dietician

Respite Care—care provided by others so family members or the primary care taker can

be relieved of the responsibi-
lities of care for a
designated period of time
RN—registered nurse
RNC—registered nurse
holding national certification
in a specialty area in nursing
RR—respiratory rate or
recovery room
RT—respiratory therapist
Rx—prescription or treatment
S & A—sugar and acetone (in
urine)
SC—subcutaneous
SCN—special care nursery
SICU—surgical intensive care
unit
Sol—solution
Spec—specimen
SSE—soap suds enema
STAT—immediately
Statistician—one who
systematically collects,
analyzes, and interprets data;
in the context of health care
services, these data are
frequently morbidity, mortality,
and vital statistics (births,
deaths)
T—temperature

Teds—elastic stockings
Telemetry—cardiac monitoring
Third-Party Payer—
reimbursement for health
services provided to a
consumer by a health
insurance company or
government program
TID—three times a day
TPN—total parenteral
nutrition
TPR—temperature, pulse,
respiration
Triage—a sorting or
prioritizing of need for better
provision of health care
delivery
Ultrasound—using high
frequency sound waves to
produce an image on an organ
or tissue in the body
VNA—visiting nurse
association
VNS—visiting nurse service
Void—urinate
VS—vital signs; temperature,
pulse, respiration, blood
pressure
WBC—white blood count
WC—wheelchair

REFERENCES

McGraw-Hill nursing dictionary (1979). New York: McGraw-Hill.
Miller, B.F. & Kline, C.B. (1983). *Encyclopedia and dictionary of medicine, nursing, and allied health,* 3rd ed. Philadelphia: Saunders.
Thomas, C.L., ed. (1985). *Taber's cyclopedic medical dictionary,* 15th ed. Philadelphia: F.A. Davis.

Bibliography

Asperheim, M.A. & Eisenhauer, L.A. (1981). *The pharmacologic basis of patient care,* 4th ed. Philadelphia: Saunders.
Atkinson, D. & Murray, M.E. (1983). *Understanding the nursing process.* New York: Macmillan.
Bates, B. (1983). *A guide to physical examination,* 3rd ed. Philadelphia: Lippincott.
Beland, K.H. & Wells, M.A. (1984). *Clinical nursing procedures.* Monterey, California: Wadsworth.
Benner, P. (1984). *From novice to expert.* Menlo Park, California: Addison-Wesley.
Corbett, J.V. (1982). *Laboratory tests in nursing practice.* East Norwalk, Connecticut: Appleton-Century-Crofts.
Corbett, J.V. (1983). *Diagnostic procedures in nursing practice.* East Norwalk, Connecticut: Appleton-Century-Crofts.
Duke University Hospital Nursing Services (1983). *Guidelines for nursing care: process and outcome.* Philadelphia: Lippincott.
Eisenhauer, L.A. & Gerald, M.C. (1984). *The nurses' 1984–85 guide to drug therapy.* Englewood Cliffs, New Jersey: Prentice-Hall.
Eschleman, M.M. (1984). *Introductory nutrition and diet therapy.* Philadelphia: Lippincott.
Fishbach, F.T.A. (1984). *A manual of laboratory diagnostic tests,* 2nd ed. Philadelphia: Lippincott.
Garb, S. (1976). *Laboratory tests in common use.* New York: Springer.

Gordon, M. (1985). *Manual of nursing diagnosis 1984–1985.* New York: McGraw-Hill.

Gordon, M. (1982). *Nursing diagnosis process and application.* New York: McGraw-Hill.

Govoni, L.E. & Hayes, J.E. (1985). *Drugs and nursing implications,* 5th ed. East Norwalk, Connecticut: Appleton-Century-Crofts.

Griffith, J.W. & Christensen, P.J. (1982). *Nursing process: application of theories, frameworks and models.* St. Louis: Mosby.

Hawkins, J.W. & Higgins, L.P. (1985). *Nursing and the American health care delivery system,* 2nd ed. New York: Tiresias.

Howe, J., Dickason, E.J., Jones, D.A. & Snider, M.J. (1984). *The handbook of nursing.* New York: Wiley.

Hui, Y.H. (1983). *Human nutrition and diet therapy.* Monterey, California: Wadsworth.

Jonas, S., ed. (1981). *Health care delivery in the United States.* New York: Springer.

Jones, D.A., Lepley, M.K. & Baker, B.A. (1984). *Health assessment across the life span.* New York: McGraw-Hill.

Kee, J.L. & Tang, H.L. (1982). *Laboratory and diagnostic tests with nursing implications.* East Norwalk, Connecticut: Appleton-Century-Crofts.

Kemp, B. & Pillitteri, A. (1984). *Fundamentals of nursing a framework for practice.* Boston: Little, Brown.

Krozier, B. & Erb, G. (1984). *Procedures supplement for fundamentals of nursing,* 2nd ed. Reading, Massachusetts: Addison-Wesley.

Laufman, H., ed. (1981). *Hospital special-care facilities.* New York: Academic Press.

Luke, B. (1984). *Principles of nutrition and diet therapy.* Boston: Little, Brown.

Malasanos, L. (1981). *Health assessment,* 2nd ed. St. Louis: Mosby.

Maram, G., Flynn, K., Abaravich, W. & Carey, S. (1976). *Cost-effectiveness of primary and team nursing.* Wakefield, Mass.: Contemporary.

Maram, G., Schlegel, M.W. & Bevis, E.O. (1974). *Primary nursing: a model for individualized care.* St. Louis: Mosby.

Mayer, G.G. (1982). *The middle manager in primary nursing.* New York: Springer.

Mayers, M.G. (1983). *A systematic approach for the nursing care plan.* New York: Appleton-Century-Crofts.

Minor, M.A.D. & Minor, S.D. (1984). *Patient care skills: positioning, range of motion, transfers, wheelchairs, and ambulation.* Reston, Virginia: Reston.

Nierenberg, J. & Janovic, F. (1978). *The hospital experience.* Indianapolis: Bobbs-Merrill.

Pagana, K.D. & Pagana, T.J. (1982). *Diagnostic testing and nursing implications.* St. Louis: Mosby.

Pascarelli, E.F., ed. (1982). *Hospital-based ambulatory care.* New York: Appleton-Century-Crofts.

Potter, P. & Perry, A. (1985). *Fundamentals of nursing.* St. Louis: Mosby.

Roemer, M.I. (1982). *An introduction to the U.S. health care system.* New York: Springer.

Rosenthal, C.J., Marshall, V.W., Macpherson, A.S., & French, S.E. (1980). *Nurses, patients, and families.* New York: Springer.

Scherer, J.C., ed. (1985). *Lippincott's nurses' drug manual.* Philadelphia: Lippincott.

Smith, S.F. (1982). *Nursing skills and evaluation.* Los Altos, California: National Nursing Review.

Sorenson, K.C. & Luckmann, J. (1979). *Basic nursing: a psychophysiologic approach.* Philadelphia: Saunders.

Spiegel, A.D. (1983). *Home health care: home birthing to hospice care.* Owings Mills, Maryland: National Health Publishing.

Suitor, C.J.W. & Crowley, M.F. (1984). *Nutrition: principles and application in health promotion,* 2nd ed. Philadelphia: Lippincott.

Suitor, C.J.W. & Crowley, M.F. (1984). *The Nutrition Workbook.* Philadelphia: Lippincott.

Thompson, J.M., McFarland, G.K., Hirsch, J.E., Tucker, S.M., & Bowers, A.C. (1985). *Clinical nursing.* St. Louis: Mosby.

Wieczorek, R.R. (1984). *Power, politics, and policy in nursing.* New York: Springer.

Index